THE 411 ON **DITCHING MEAT** AND **GOING VEG**

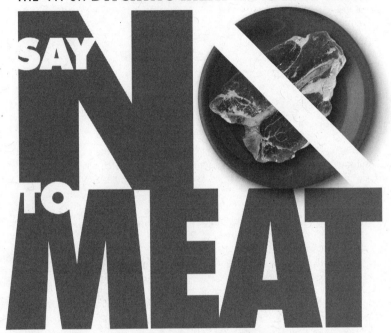

SAY NO TO MEAT

AMANDA STROMBOM AND STEWART ROSE

HEALTHY LIVING PUBLICATIONS
SUMMERTOWN, TENNESSEE

Cover and interior design: Jim Scattaregia
Illustrations: Casey McDonald, Jessica Dadds and Edwina Cusolito

Healthy Living Publications, an imprint of Book Publishing Company
P.O. Box 99
Summertown, TN 38483
888-260-8458
www.bookpubco.com

ISBN: 978-1-57067-265-1

Printed in Canada

17 16 15 14 13 12 11   9 8 7 6 5 4 3 2 1

The information in this book is for educational purposes only. The information is not intended as a substitute for a physician's diagnosis and care. The authors urge everyone, including those with medical problems or symptoms, to consult a licensed physician before undertaking any lifestyle or medical changes.

Library of Congress Cataloging-in-Publication Data

Strombom, Amanda.
  Say no to meat! : the 411 on ditching meat and going veg /
Amanda Strombom and Stewart Rose.
     p. cm.
  Includes index.
  ISBN 978-1-57067-265-1
  1. Vegetarianism. I. Rose, Stewart D., 1956- II. Title.
  RM236.S77 2011
  613.2'62--dc22

2011005772

Printed on recycled paper

Book Publishing Company is a member of Green Press Initiative. We chose to print this title on paper with 100% post consumer recycled content, processed without chlorine, which saved the following natural resources:

17 trees
482 pounds of solid waste
7,938 gallons of water
1,648 pounds of greenhouse gases
5 million BTU of energy

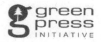

For more information on Green Press Initiative, visit www.greenpressinitiative.org. Environmental impact estimates were made using the Environmental Defense Fund Paper Calculator. For more information visit www.edf.org/papercalculator.

For **Matthew** and **Emma Strombom**, **Talia Helman**,
and a new generation of young vegetarians.

Contents

Acknowledgments

A big thank you! Thanks to our publisher, Healthy Living Publications, for all their help and guidance. You guys really rock! We also thank Jo Stepaniak and Cheryl Redmond for a great job on the copy editing, and Jim Scattaregia for the fantastic cover design and interior layout. Thanks also to Edwina Cusolito, Casey McDonald, and Jessica Dadds for the cool illustrations. Most of all we thank Doug and Susan for their love and support. Finally, we wish to thank the members and supporters of Vegetarians of Washington, and all the young vegetarians who inspired us to write this book by asking so many questions!

CHAPTER 1

The Basics

What's this book about?

I'll bet you have at least one friend, or you've met at least one person, who says he or she is a vegetarian. Becoming a vegetarian is not only way cool, it's also a very smart move.

It seems like more and more people are curious to learn what being a vegetarian is all about. We call these people the veg-curious. Whether you're veg-curious, or you're already a vegetarian but want to learn more about it, this book is for you.

Becoming a vegetarian is easier than you think. While there are a few things you should know, becoming a vegetarian is not rocket science. This book will tell you everything you need to know to get started, and we'll give it to you straight. You'll learn about the many advantages of being a vegetarian, and we'll explain how to go totally vegetarian. You'll also find advice on how to handle friends, parents, teachers, and ministers. You'll get some great starter recipes for dishes that taste outrageously good.

There's an old Chinese proverb that says that every journey starts with but a single step. For many of you, this book will be the first step on your journey to becoming a vegetarian. Few people become vegetarians overnight. It's a step-by-step process. Every time you make a vegetarian food choice, you are one step closer to improving your health, saving the animals, and sustaining the environment. OK, let's get started.

I'm confused. What exactly is a vegetarian?

A vegetarian is someone who eats no meat, poultry, or fish products. There are several subsets of this:

> ➤ A lacto-ovo vegetarian eats dairy and egg products, but avoids all meat, poultry, and fish.
> ➤ A lacto-vegetarian eats dairy but avoids egg products as well as meat, poultry, and fish.

> An ovo-vegetarian eats eggs but avoids dairy products as well as meat, poultry, and fish.

> A vegan or total vegetarian eats no animal products—no meat, poultry, fish, dairy, or eggs. Many vegans also avoid eating honey.

What about people who eat fish, or even meat just once in a while?

Sorry, we can't bend the rules. A person who still eats fish is really a pesco-vegetarian or a pescatarian. A person who mostly eats plant foods, but will still eat a little meat occasionally, is usually called a flexitarian. While both pescatarians and flexitarians have taken a big step in the right direction, they still have to go the whole nine yards if they want to call themselves vegetarians.

How many vegetarians are there?

If you become a vegetarian you'll be in good company. A 2008 poll conducted for the magazine *Vegetarian Times* showed that 3.2 percent of U.S. adults, or 7.3 million Americans, are vegetarians, and an additional 10 percent, or 22.8 million, eat a mostly vegetarian diet.

Remember that although there have been vegetarians throughout history, many people are only now discovering the benefits of a vegetarian diet, and are starting to make changes in what they eat. Some estimates put the number of people who have tried vegetarian foods, such as veggie burgers, from time to time to be as high as 40 percent of the population.

There are plenty of vegetarians around the world. The countries where following a vegetarian diet is even more popular than it is here include India, where 30 percent of the population follows a vegetarian diet; Israel, where 10 percent are vegetarian; Great Britain, with 5 percent; and the Netherlands, with 4.4 percent.

Is it hard to find vegetarian food?

In most cities, you'll be amazed at how easy it is to be vegetarian today. Almost all major grocery stores, and many of the smaller ones, carry veggie burgers and other meat alternatives, tofu, and soymilk, along with all the fruits, vegetables, beans, nuts, seeds, and grains that make up a wholesome vegetarian diet. If you like to eat out, you'll find veggie options in most restaurants, so there's no need to fear that you'll be left with nothing to eat. If you live in a small town, there may be fewer veggie choices available on the menu, but remember you can always ask the chef to make you something special, or just hold the meat. It's so worth it!

Do I have to change my politics to become a vegetarian?

Don't be lead astray by political stereotypes about vegetarians. Vegetarianism is definitely bipartisan. You don't have to change your politics to become a vegetarian. You can belong to any political party (or no political party); you can be ultraconservative or super liberal. In fact, vegetarians are well represented among both Democrats and Republicans. For instance, Matthew Scully, who was President George W. Bush's chief speechwriter, is a vegetarian and author of an important animal rights book, *Dominion*, while Democratic congressman Dennis Kucinich is an outspoken vegan. Politics can be very divisive and distracting when it comes to becoming a vegetarian. So just keep your focus on the food, and don't get lost in the wilderness of American politics.

Will following a vegetarian diet go against my religion?

Put your soul at ease. Being a vegetarian is completely allowable in all the major religions of the world. In fact, in many religions, vegetarianism has a rich history that is surprising to many people. To learn more about how easily following a vegetarian diet fits in with different religions, see page 61.

Can you name some vegetarians I may have heard of?

We've got bragging rights. Vegetarians have been found among the ranks of geniuses such as Albert Einstein, founding fathers such as Benjamin Franklin, humanitarians such as Mahatma Gandhi, Olympic gold medalists such as Carl Lewis, military commanders such as British air chief marshal Hugh Dowding, gifted musicians such as Paul McCartney of the Beatles, talented actors such as Tobey Maguire (who played Spiderman), and great men of faith such as the founder of the Salvation Army, William Booth.

There are so many vegetarians, it's hard to know who to include. We've picked a selection of those you may have heard of. To see a more complete list, go to www.ivu.org/people or www.peta2.com. Remember that the list of famous vegetarians is changing all the time, as more people decide to go veggie.

Historical and Well-Known Figures

Susan B. Anthony, American suffragist and civil rights leader

William Booth, founder of the Salvation Army

Charles Darwin, British naturalist
who first proposed the theory of evolution

Leonardo da Vinci, artist and scientist

Thomas Edison, inventor of the electric light bulb

Albert Einstein, physicist who devised the theory of relativity

Benjamin Franklin, a founding father of the United States

Mahatma Gandhi, Indian civil rights leader

Gustav Holst, classical composer

Abraham Kook, first chief rabbi of Israel

Gustav Mahler, classical composer

Isaac Newton, English mathematician who formulated
the theory of gravitation and laws of motion

Plato, Greek philosopher

Pythagoras, Greek mathematician

Albert Schweitzer, physician and theologian
who won the Nobel Peace Prize

Coretta Scott King and **Dexter Scott King**,
wife and son of **Martin Luther King**

Socrates, Greek philosopher

John Wesley, founder of the Methodist Church

Ellen G. White, founder of the Seventh-day Adventist Church

Present-Day Musicians

Paula Abdul, American singer, choreographer, TV personality

Bryan Adams, Canadian singer

André Benjamin (André 3000), American rapper

Tom Higgenson, lead singer of Plain White T's

Andy Hurley, drummer with Fall Out Boy

Anthony Kiedis, lead singer of the Red Hot Chili Peppers

Avril Lavigne, Canadian singer

Leona Lewis, British singer

Travis Miguel, guitarist with Atreyu

Moby, American singer and instrumentalist

Jason Mraz, American singer-songwriter

Paul McCartney, lead singer of the Beatles

Prince, American singer-songwriter

Shania Twain, Canadian singer

Carrie Underwood, American singer

Present-Day Actors and Entertainers
(and their current and well-known movies or shows)

Penelope Cruz, *Nine, Vanilla Sky*

Ellen DeGeneres, *The Ellen DeGeneres Show*

Emily Deschanel, *Bones*

Michael J. Fox, *Back to the Future*

Ginnifer Goodwin, *He's Just Not That Into You*

Woody Harrelson, *Zombieland*

Dustin Hoffman, *Rainman, Hook*

Tobey Maguire, *Spiderman*

Hayden Panettiere, *Heroes*

Natalie Portman, *Star Wars, Black Swan*

Alicia Silverstone, *Silence Becomes You, Clueless*

Kristen Wiig, *Saturday Night Live*

Athletes

Hank Aaron, baseball player; former home run record holder

Desmond Howard, former NFL wide receiver, Super Bowl MVP

Georges Laraque, former right wing for the Montreal Canadiens

Carl Lewis, track and field athlete,
winner of nine Olympic gold medals

Bode Miller, alpine ski racer;
Olympic gold medalist and World Cup champion

John Salley, basketball player; four-time NBA champion

Dave Scott, triathlete; won six Ironman World Championship events

Ed Templeton, champion skateboarder

Jamie Thomas, champion skateboarder

Ricky Williams, running back for the Miami Dolphins

Can you give me one good reason why I should go vegetarian?

Actually we can give you more than one good reason to go vegetarian. Going veggie is a popular thing to do these days, and people have all kinds of reasons for doing so, but most fall within five categories:

> ➤ If you care deeply about animals, you should stop eating them so that they won't have to endure harsh conditions on factory-style farms and then die just to produce food for us.

> ➤ If you are concerned about saving the environment, giving up eating meat is the single most important action you can take to help reduce global warming, reduce water pollution, and save resources for future generations.

> ➤ If you worry about all the world's hungry people, raising livestock is so wasteful of food, that you'd be making a lot more food available for hungry people by giving up eating animal products.

> ➤ If you care about eating more healthfully, to avoid the many diseases associated with eating meat, or just to feel better right now, going vegetarian is the best way to live a long and healthy life.

> ➤ And if you are spiritually inclined, choosing to go vegetarian can be an important part of your spiritual practices and beliefs.

All these reasons are good reasons. While some people are motivated to become vegetarians for just one reason, others become vegetarians for a combination of reasons. The good news is that not only do they all work well, but they all work well together.

You can learn more about the various reasons for going vegetarian by reading the answers to the questions in the chapters about health, the animals, the environment, global hunger, and the spirit. The more you learn about it, the more you'll discover what a great idea it is to go vegetarian.

What's wrong with meat, fish, dairy, and eggs?

There's plenty wrong with animal food products; in fact, they cause so many problems that they should come with warning labels, like cigarettes do: "Caution: eating meat will damage your health, and producing it pollutes the world and makes animals suffer, all for no good reason!"

Eating meat, fish, dairy, and eggs has been found to increase the risk of heart disease, many cancers, stroke, diabetes, and many other serious diseases. They have also been found to have links to health issues as wide-ranging as acne, asthma, poor concentration, and menstrual cramps.

The raising of animals for food causes untold damage to the environment, including contributing significantly to water pollution, ecological destruction, and global warming. The animals themselves don't have a good experience either, as they usually are raised in factory farms where no thought is given to their welfare.

It may also surprise you to learn that feeding our crops to farm animals is very wasteful. In fact, if the United States alone became a vegetarian nation, we'd easily have enough extra food to feed all the hungry people in the world. You can learn more about all these problems in the relevant chapters of this book.

Why is so much information on vegetarian diets contradictory?

Are you confused? One moment you hear this and the next you hear that. There's a blizzard of information available to us these days, and much of it is contradictory. No wonder half the country doesn't know which end is up when it comes to food and nutrition issues in general. The reasons for the confusion depend on the source of the information and the goals of the person who has written it. Much of the information out there is of very low quality, containing nothing but misconceptions and outright deceptions. However, when you get your information from a steady diet of high-quality sources, the picture becomes much clearer.

Always bear in mind the example of cigarettes. It wasn't so long ago that doctors were advertising which brand of cigarettes they smoked, even though the truth about the dangers of smoking had been known for many years. Since the surgeon general first announced that cigarettes can damage your health, it has taken more than fifty years to get to the point where cigarette smoking is banned in most public places. Changing public opinion takes time, especially when the public really doesn't want to change. See chapter 7 for more information on this subject.

What are the different sources of information on nutrition?

To help you find your way through the forest we've identified the problems with some of the most common sources of nutritional information. Let's go through them one by one:

Advertisements and Packaging

Advertising rules! For many of us, the only nutrition information we receive is through advertisements on the television or radio, in magazines, or on the packaging of food in the store. The ads and packaging are paid for by companies wanting to promote their products, so they make every possible effort to convince you that their products are nutritious, tasty, and necessary for your happiness. To do this, they use all kinds of tricks. For example, meat advertisers will tell you about the protein in meat, implying that it's good for you, while leaving out mention of all the cholesterol and saturated fat. Remember who benefits from the sale of this product and focus on the information required by law—the nutrition facts label and the list of ingredients.

News Reports

Don't believe everything you read in the papers. The newspapers are not nonprofits. They're in business to make money. They do this by gaining circulation (the number of people reading the paper). The greater the circulation, the more they can charge for advertisements, and selling advertisements is how newspapers make most of their money.

To get you to buy their paper in the first place, they need to catch your eye. Two common methods of doing this are to tell you something that's the opposite of what's expected or to shock you with over-sensationalized reports. A story about a man who lived to be ninety while smoking two packs of cigarettes a day would be an example of a story that is the opposite of what you would expect, and is therefore very eye-catching. A visit to the cancer ward in your local hospital would tell a very different story. It would tell a story of smokers suffering from cancer, and then all too often dying before their time was due. The better newspapers and television news reports may give you the rest of the story at the end of the article or the newscast. They will tell you that the man who smoked two packs a day and lived to be ninety years old is an exception, and that most smokers die young. But many reporters won't.

Another reason for not telling you the truth, or the whole truth, is that many news organizations fear offending their advertisers. Food companies advertise widely, so papers may avoid reporting the disadvantages of certain animal products to ensure that those industries continue to support them. This is particularly true of the free magazines you find in natural food stores.

Are there really always two legitimate sides to every story? A misplaced sense of the need for balance can make a news report very confusing. When reporting, journalists often feel that they need to present both sides of an issue. This is appropriate where opinions are concerned, in politics for example. But where facts are involved, providing "balance" by reporting on someone crazy, ignorant, or dishonest enough to deny the facts leaves the reader confused as to what the truth really is. For instance, scientists and doctors have determined time and again that plant foods provide all the protein a person needs. It's been proven so many times that you would think that no one would question it. However, when a journalist quotes a scientific study showing that plant proteins are more than adequate, they will then often include a quote from an unreliable source that says meat is necessary for protein, just to include what's called balance. This gives the reader the false impression that both sides have an equal chance at being right. This practice, aimed at providing a misplaced notion of political correctness and fairness, creates confusion. The problem is that in doing this they are not being fair to the facts. While people are entitled to their own opinions they are not entitled to their own facts, and it's the facts that should drive the content of news stories about health, and not balance.

The bottom line is this. Whenever a news story catches your eye, try to look beyond the headlines and all the sensationalism. Look for other reliable sources of information to see what they say on the topic, and always remember to read the article all the way through to the end. The article may not actually say what the headline implies.

Websites

Websites covering food and nutrition issues can be divided up into the good, the bad, and the ugly. Unfortunately, the good are few, the bad are many, and even the ugly are numerous.

Websites are quick and easy to find via a search engine, but they are also quick and easy to create, so anyone can put information on the Internet and it can be difficult to determine whether it is true or not. It can be even harder to determine just who is really behind a website and what their real agenda may be.

But all is not lost. We've collected a list of websites that provide reliable and easy-to-access information on page 167. Stick with these and you should do fine.

Talk Shows

Talk shows are about entertainment, not education. The information on these shows, sometimes called infotainment, is often not reliable. Many people are excited about movie stars and celebrities, but they forget that they really know no more about most subjects than the rest of us. Talk shows are fine if you have a few hours to kill, but not for learning about food and nutrition.

Medical Studies

In news reports, on websites, and even on talk shows, you will hear medical studies mentioned, to prove the point they are trying to make. The implication is that if a medical study indicates something, it must be true. While good-quality medical studies are vital for determining the truth, some medical studies are biased, poorly carried out, or just made up.

One way to determine whether mention of a medical study is reliable is to see if a reference is provided, detailing where the study was published. You can also google the title of a study and see where it was published. Make sure that it was published in a peer-reviewed journal, such as the *American Journal of Cardiology* or the *Journal of the American Medical Association.* While such a study, written in scientific terms, can be very hard for the average person to understand, just knowing that it does exist, and that a respected journal reviewed and published it, can provide some reassurance.

Books

A good book is worth its weight in gold. One advantage of a book is that much more space is available to explain specific topics in detail, so it can give a much fuller picture than a website, magazine article or news report. It costs time and money to publish a book, and to have it distributed to bookstores and libraries, which can put off all but the most dedicated writers, so books tend to be more reliable sources of information.

That being said, there are still many books in circulation not worth the paper they're printed on. However, we've assembled a reliable bibliography on page 167, listing some quality books that you can depend on.

Why should I believe this book?

We rolled up our sleeves and went where the facts took us. To write this book, and its sister book, *The Vegetarian Solution* by Stewart Rose, we went back to the source material. We read the many medical and other scientific studies on how a vegetarian diet affects our health and the environment in particular, and drew clear conclusions from the most reliable studies. The information given in this book is based on those studies, so you can rest assured that reliable scientific research shows time and again that a vegetarian diet is beneficial to our health and the environment. You can feel comfortable in knowing that by going vegetarian, you are doing the right thing for your health, for the animals, for the environment, and for your spirit.

How is this book different from other vegetarian books?

We give it to you straight and we don't play games. This book is not written to shock or outrage you, or even just convince you that it's cool to be a vegetarian, since we don't believe that such tricks will help you stay vegetarian for long. The facts and issues discussed are presented with the goal of helping you make smart decisions and lifestyle choices. If you value life, health, compassion, charity, and protecting the environment, you will soon see that choosing vegetarian food is the right thing to do.

As with any major change in society, myths and doubts persist. In this book, the myths, doubts, and questions about vegetarian food and diets are all discussed, and full explanations of what's really going on are given. The information is provided in an easy question and answer format, so that you can quickly find the information you are looking for. In this way, we hope to give you the confidence to ask for the food you want to eat.

However, information is not enough. The proof is in the pudding. That's why we've included a section explaining how to use foods that may be new to you, such as tofu, tempeh, and quinoa. Then we follow it up with a great selection of recipes.

This book is intended as an introduction, to get you started. If you want to learn more about a particular topic, see the selection of books and websites provided in the Resources section (page 167). Anyone can become a vegetarian with just a little knowledge and skill. We'll answer all your questions and help you get started!

CHAPTER 2

For Your Health

How much does food matter to my health?

Food is number one. The top causes of death—heart attacks, strokes, and most cancers—are all related to diet. So are most of the other major health challenges of modern life, such as diabetes and Alzheimer's disease. The food we choose to eat is usually the single most important factor in determining our health and how long we live.

J. Wayne McFarland, MD, former fellow of the Mayo Clinic, gives it to you straight: "Food has to do with the very essence of life itself. It is the fuel that maintains, repairs, and runs the human machine. It is the source of the material needed to keep the body tissue healthy, vigorous, and free of sickness."

It's a fact of life. Don't let anyone tell you otherwise. Genetics account for only a very small percentage of disease. Pollution is a bad thing, but doesn't cause even a small fraction of the disease that unhealthy food choices cause. Couch potatoes arise, start walking more and driving less. Your body will thank you for it, but not nearly as much as it will thank you for a vegetarian diet. By all means get your vaccinations, but no vaccine can give you any measure of protection from the leading causes of death in America. Only a healthy vegetarian diet can do that.

Are you sure that being a vegetarian is safe?

Rest assured, the finest medical authorities have confirmed time and again that vegetarian and vegan diets are safe. In fact, given all the evidence we have about the negative health effects of meat and other animal products, a better question would be to ask how anyone could think that a meat-centered diet is safe! If you still have any doubts, here is the American Dietetic Association stamp of approval:

It is the position of the American Dietetic Association that appropriately planned vegetarian diets, including total vegetarian or vegan diets, are healthful, nutritionally adequate, and may provide health benefits in the prevention and treatment of certain diseases. Well-planned vegetarian diets are appropriate for individuals during all stages of the life cycle, including pregnancy, lactation, infancy, childhood, and adolescence, and for athletes.

Is a vegetarian diet better for my health?

The evidence is in: vegetarian, and especially vegan, diets are much better for your health than meat-centered diets. Marion Nestle, professor of nutrition at New York University, says, "There is no question that vegetarian diets are as healthy as you can get. The evidence is so strong and overwhelming, and produced over such a long period of time, that it's no longer debatable."

Don't let the absence of technology fool you. Vegetarian food is simple yet powerful. Modern medical studies show time and again that a vegetarian diet is the best way to reduce your risk of many of the common diseases currently plaguing our society, such as heart disease, stroke, cancer, and diabetes. It also forms a valuable part of the treatment for these diseases. The American Dietetic Association says, "Vegetarian diets are often associated with a number of health advantages, including lower blood cholesterol levels, lower risk of heart disease, lower blood pressure levels, and lower risk of hypertension and type 2 diabetes. Vegetarians tend to have a lower body mass index (BMI) and lower overall cancer rates."

You won't have to wait long to experience the health benefits of a vegetarian diet. Not only does a vegetarian diet help prevent serious chronic diseases, it can also help improve aspects of your health right now. For instance, studies show that menstrual cramps and acne are less severe for vegetarians than others. Better nutrition can even help your performance in school.

You can really go the distance on a vegetarian diet. For his book *Eat to Live*, Joel Fuhrman, MD, analyzed medical studies and found that people who follow a vegetarian diet for at least half their life live, on average, thirteen years longer than others. They wouldn't be living so much longer if they were missing something in their diet!

There's just one thing. To get the greatest health benefit from a vegetarian diet, go easy on the junk food. You can certainly have treats once in a while with no problem. But a steady diet of cola and fries is not the best way to go. See page 107 for healthier snack ideas.

Aren't our bodies designed to eat meat?

Just ask yourself this question: Can you or anyone you know run out into a field, chase down a cow, and with nothing but your teeth and your fingernails, kill it, cut through its hide, and eat its meat raw? Do you know anyone who can even chase down a squirrel? Now ask yourself this question: Do you know anybody who can't pull a carrot out of the ground or an apple off a tree? The only way we can eat meat is because we have developed tools and weapons to do for us what our bodies could never do on their own. While we can use our brains to obtain all kinds of unnatural foods, our health is best when we follow a more natural diet.

The fact is that the human being is designed to be an herbivore (a plant eater), but many people think that we are omnivores (creatures that can eat animal or plant foods). Don't just take our word for it. Here's what William Clifford Roberts, MD, editor in chief of the *American Journal of Cardiology* has to say: "Although we think we are one, and we act as if we are one, human beings are not natural carnivores. When we kill animals to eat them, they end up killing us because their flesh, which contains cholesterol and saturated fat, was never intended for human beings, who are natural herbivores."

It may take some time to get used to the idea of humans being natural herbivores, but if you compare our anatomy and physiology to those of carnivores (meat-eating animals), such as cats, and to omnivores, such as dogs or bears, you'll see that we are quite different. Our back teeth are flatter for grinding, our front teeth are small for nibbling, our finger nails are more like hooves than claws, and our intestines are ten to twelve times our body length, just like many other herbivores such as gorillas, elephants, horses, and sheep. True carnivores and omnivores all have intestines that are only four to six times their body length, quite different from ours. Take a look at the chart on page 24 for comparison.

Just to make sure, medical researchers conducted an experiment where they fed meat to different animals. Despite being given huge amounts of meat, dogs and cats never got clogged arteries. But when an herbivore such as a rabbit was given meat regularly, it started to develop clogged arteries in a very short time. By comparing our bodies to those of carnivores and omnivores, and by observing the effect meat has on our bodies, we can see that we were not designed to eat meat.

Will a vegetarian diet help me lose weight?

You can win the battle of the bulge. Vegetarians, and especially vegans, tend to be slimmer than meat eaters. Medical studies have shown that vegetarians have a much lower risk of obesity compared with nonvegetarians. While just becoming a vegetarian won't automatically make you as thin as a rail, it does give you a definite advantage.

Anatomy and Physiology Comparisons

Carnivores

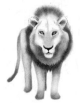

Incisor Teeth: Short pointed
Molar Teeth: Sharp
Nails: Sharp claws
Saliva: No digestive enzymes
Stomach Acid: pH of 1 with food in stomach
Small Intestine: 3–6 times body length
Urine: Extremely concentrated
Perspires Through Skin Pores: No

Omnivores

Incisor Teeth: Short pointed
Molar Teeth: Sharp
Nails: Sharp claws
Saliva: No digestive enzymes
Stomach Acid: pH of 1 with food in stomach
Small Intestine: 4–6 times body length
Urine: Extremely concentrated
Perspires Through Skin Pores: No

Herbivores

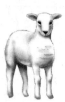

Incisor Teeth: Broad and flattened
Molar Teeth: Flattened
Nails: Flattened nails, hooves
Saliva: Carbohydrate digesting enzymes
Stomach Acid: pH of 4–5 with food in stomach
Small Intestine: 10–12 times body length
Urine: Moderately concentrated
Perspires Through Skin Pores: Yes

Humans

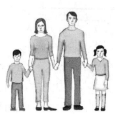

Incisor Teeth: Broad and flattened
Molar Teeth: Flattened
Nails: Flattened nails
Saliva: Carbohydrate digesting enzymes
Stomach Acid: pH of 4–5 with food in stomach
Small Intestine: 10–11 times body length
Urine: Moderately concentrated
Perspires Through Skin Pores: Yes

Figure 1. Carnivores, herbivores, and omnivores have different physical characteristics.

Animal products are just too intense. In general, they pack more calories per ounce than plant foods, and they have no fiber, so you have to eat more calories before you feel full. When you cut out animal foods, and replace them with high-fiber foods such as fruits, vegetables, legumes, and whole grains, you'll find that you feel full sooner, and gain less weight, because plant foods generally have more bulk and fewer calories.

Quality matters too; beware of junk foods. Junk foods contain very little in the way of nutrients, hence they are often said to contain "empty calories", whereas unprocessed plant foods are very rich in nutrients such as vitamins and minerals. Our bodies can recognize when we have eaten the nutrients we need, and they send a signal to the brain to indicate that we've had enough. When you eat junk foods that signal gets delayed. Many people pig out on junk foods when they are stressed. Don't make this mistake. Find other ways of dealing with the stresses of life.

The formula is simple. A healthful vegetarian diet, made up of fruits, vegetables, whole grains, beans, and nuts, supplies plenty of nutrients and helps us to feel full sooner, so it discourages overeating and supports us in maintaining a healthy weight. Avoiding dairy and eggs results in even better weight control, since these foods are often high in fat or prepared in ways that make them high in fat.

Girls, skip the catwalk. Deciding to go vegetarian with the aim of looking like a fashion model is not a good idea. Fashion models are required to look unhealthily skinny by some magazines and their example is not a good one to follow. Some people are obsessed with fashion, and obsessions can cause a person to lose sight of the real goal of being a healthy, happy person. You may not be skinny as a rail, but who cares? You'll be a healthier and happier person knowing that you're eating foods that are good for you, for the animals, for the world's hungry, and for the planet, than by trying to starve yourself.

Will a vegetarian diet help clear up my acne?

Skin care manufacturers would like you to believe that the only way to reduce acne is to buy their expensive products and to use them on your skin day and night. But you'll probably find that lack of blemishes and clarity of skin are determined far more by what you eat than by what products you put on your skin. Your skin is the largest organ in your body, so it makes sense to take care of it by eating the right foods.

Folklore tells us to avoid certain foods such as chocolate to avoid acne, but it seems that it's more important to focus on getting good nutrition all around. An Australian study published in the *American Journal of Clinical Nutrition* showed that in only twelve weeks, boys aged fifteen to twenty-five had a 50 percent reduction in the amount of their acne when they were fed a diet higher in whole grains, fruits, vegetables, and legumes, compared with a control group who continued to eat their usual high-fat and high-sugar "junk food" diet. Researchers at Harvard School of Public Health found a strong correlation between a higher consumption of cow's milk and a higher occurrence of acne.

Attack your pimples from the inside out. What's good for your body as a whole is also going to be good for your skin, so try a whole-foods vegetarian diet, cutting out dairy products and junk food in particular, and you could find that your skin improves in just a few weeks.

Will a vegetarian diet help me concentrate better?

Those veggies can make you sharp. A diet based on natural whole foods, such as a balanced vegetarian diet, will help. The food we eat can make a big difference in our ability to concentrate, and in young people this is often reflected in their behavior in class.

Don't get into a crash! When you eat junk foods, your blood sugar skyrockets and then crashes. Many teachers will tell you that they can recognize when a student has eaten a lot of sugar-laden or junk foods. Some studies of people with attention deficit disorder (ADD) have shown that artificial food additives can aggravate their condition. So stay natural and stay clear of junk foods. Give your brain only the best.

Better food can make all the difference both for you and your school. At Appleton Central Alternative Charter High School in Appleton, Wisconsin, student behavior problems were so bad that the police were called in every day. Many of the students also had trouble concentrating and learning. The school decided to change the entire cafeteria menu as part of an overall program to turn the school around, so only nutritious food was served for breakfast and lunch. The vending machines were taken away—no more junk food. Since the start of the new food program, the number of students who have dropped out, been expelled, been found using drugs or carrying weapons, or who have committed suicide have all dropped to zero and grades are on the uptick. These students discovered that by eating more nutritious foods they became happier and more focused, so they are enthusiastic about the change.

A vegetarian diet may even help you avoid a life of crime. Robert King was sentenced to a twenty-eight-year term at Powhatan Correctional Center in Virginia for burglary. When he got to prison, King weighed 275 pounds and was addicted to cocaine. Since that time he has eaten his way back to physical and mental health. King became a near vegan through a special program at the prison and it had a big effect on him. King lost fifty pounds, freed himself of drug dependency, and earned fifty-three credits at J. Sargeant Reynolds Community College with an A average. King credits his new diet for his big turnaround, saying, "it all begins and ends with my diet." Corrections facility director Tom Parlett confirms the effect of the better diet on the inmates in the program and states that "their whole attitudes have changed."

So give tofu a try! If you are struggling to concentrate, and have a hard time controlling your behavior, it's likely that the food you're eating is contributing to the problem. Try switching to a nutritious vegetarian diet and watch your concentration improve.

I have asthma. Will a vegetarian diet help?

Vegetarians breathe easier. While there are many different factors that can cause asthma, the food you eat is certainly an important factor. In one study, patients were placed on a vegetarian diet, which excluded dairy and eggs. This had a big impact. In only four months, 71 percent found that their asthma improved, and after a year 92 percent had improved. In almost all cases, the improvement was so great that the patients were able to stop or substantially reduce their medication. So why not give it a try? Maybe by giving up the meat, dairy, and eggs, you'll also be able to give up using your inhaler.

I'm an athlete. Can I build muscles and endurance on a vegetarian diet?

Don't fall for the meat myth. Athletes often think that they need to eat meat to build muscles, but in fact medical studies have shown that protein from veggie sources is just as valuable for an athlete as protein from meat. Consider baseball legend Hank Aaron, Olympic gold medalist Carl Lewis, and Ironman triathlete Dave Scott, who is considered by many to be the fittest man on earth. These men all reached their peak performance on vegetarian diets, showing that a vegetarian diet is certainly no impediment, and may well have helped them achieve outstanding records. Bill Pearl, who was chosen to be Mr. Universe and Mr. America four times, and Johnny Weissmuller, the original Tarzan of movie fame, built their impressive muscles on vegetarian diets. Many other athletes have discovered that you can build both strong muscles and outstanding endurance on a vegetarian diet. For a list of famous vegetarian athletes, see page 13.

Work, not meat, makes muscles! Muscles are built by stressing them through exercise. This stimulates the muscles to use protein supplies in the blood to build up the muscles. As long as there are adequate supplies of protein in the bloodstream, you will have no trouble building muscle. For more information about protein from plant foods, see page 80.

Vegetarians have better endurance. While the protein from veggies is just as good as from meat, it has been found that a vegetarian diet is much more effective than a meat-based diet in building endurance. In a study conducted in Sweden, athletes tried three different diets, each for several weeks, with their endurance tested on each. The results showed that when athletes were eating a balanced vegetarian diet, they had three times the endurance as when they were following a meat-centered diet.

The vegan wins the race. In 1999, Scott Jurek, then twenty-five years old, became the youngest man ever to win the prestigious Western States One Hundred-Mile Endurance Run. He went on to be the only seven-time consecutive winner. What did he eat to win all those races? Scott Jurek followed a vegan diet consisting of fruits, vegetables, grains, nuts, and legumes. Other athletes have had similar results. Carl Lewis, the track and field champion, said he had his best performance ever when he went vegan.

To reach their peak performance, athletes get all of the essential ingredients by eating plenty of fruits, vegetables, grains, nuts, and legumes. According to Scott Jurek, for an athlete, just as for anyone else, it is important to eat a properly balanced diet consisting of whole plant foods in sufficient quantity in accordance with the amount of exercise you do. One of the most common mistakes athletes make is simply not eating enough. Calorie needs vary depending on the amount, intensity, and type of exercise. Even when resting, an athlete's metabolism can be up to 30 percent greater than a nonathlete's. Some athletes need over 4,000 calories per day.

Will a vegetarian diet help with my menstrual cramps?

Diet can help. Medical researchers have found that a low-fat vegetarian diet significantly reduces both the intensity and the length of menstrual cramps and PMS in most girls, so if you suffer from painful menstrual cramps every month, it is well worth trying a vegetarian diet.

Is it safe for me to be pregnant and still be vegetarian?

Study after study has shown that a vegetarian diet during pregnancy is both safe and health promoting. In fact, the American Dietetic Association says, "A vegetarian diet planned in accordance with current dietary recommendations can easily meet the nutritional needs of pregnancy."

Plan ahead. If your diet is less than ideal, and you're thinking of having a baby, or have found out that you're pregnant, now is the time to improve your diet. Look for substitutions you can make to the foods you usually eat, to increase the amounts of whole grains, beans, nuts, and seeds you eat, and especially to eat lots of fresh fruits and vegetables. Give yourself some nutritional insurance. Start taking a daily prenatal supplement right away. Having sufficient folic acid in the first three weeks of pregnancy, for example, has been found to prevent spina bifida (a very serious disease). If you wait until you discover that you are pregnant, it could be too late. Your baby deserves only the best, so go easy on junk food. The time in the womb is a vitally important time for a baby's growth and development. Don't waste it on a diet of french fries, Coke, and Twinkies.

How can being a vegetarian or vegan help protect my baby?

Plant-based diets protect your baby from a variety of toxic substances. These include pesticides, herbicides, and industrial pollutants such as mercury, dioxins, and PCBs, which have been shown to cause damage to babies' brains and nervous systems and increase the risk of several forms of cancer. Most of the exposure we get to these chemicals actually comes from animals that have stored and concentrated these chemicals in their flesh, not from plant foods. When we eat animal products, we receive their whole lifetime's accumulation of those chemicals, which can be a hundred times more concentrated than that found on the crops themselves. By eliminating meat, fish, dairy, and eggs from your diet, you are dramatically reducing both your and your baby's exposure to toxic chemicals.

Note that it's worth choosing organic foods, especially if you still eat some animal products, whenever you can, to limit your exposure to pesticides and herbicides, but industrial toxins can still be present even in organic food.

After your baby is born you may wish to breast-feed. If you do, you'll want to produce the most wholesome breast milk possible. This means avoiding exposure to toxic chemicals, which can make their way into your breast milk. Researchers at the Michigan School of Public Health discovered that women's breast milk had PCB levels twice that which would be legal in commercial dairy milk. The problem of toxins in breast milk is a problem that has been brushed aside by many breast-feeding advocates, but it deserves your attention. The good news is that vegetarian women have much lower levels of environmental contaminants such as DDT, DDE, and PCBs in their breast milk, compared to the breast milk of women in the general population. Breast-feeding has many valuable benefits for your baby, so the important thing to do is to cut out eating animal products as soon as possible, to limit the accumulation of these chemicals in your body.

If you choose not to breast-feed, or when you stop, consider using a soy-based formula instead of a cow's milk formula. Cow's milk has higher levels of both agricultural and industrial toxins, has been linked to juvenile diabetes, and is loaded with saturated fat and cholesterol. Soy-based formulas have none of these disadvantages, and have been used safely for a more than a hundred years.

Don't I need to drink milk to have strong bones?

Just ask yourself this question: Can you think of one other animal that consumes milk past the age of weaning? Now ask yourself what other animal consumes the milk of another species? The answer is none.

For generations, milk has been promoted as a natural food, and in recent years, emphasis has been put on the fact that milk contains calcium. It is therefore assumed that milk helps to build stronger bones and prevent osteoporosis. But women in Asia and Africa, who rarely or never drink milk, don't get osteoporosis as often as American women, and in fact no studies have found any evidence of improved bone density from consuming more dairy products. The reason for this is explained on page 83.

Where do you think the cow got its calcium to give to you anyway? From plants of course! It also turns out that the calcium in most veggies is even better absorbed than from milk. Good sources of calcium include vegetables such as kale, collard greens, bok choy, and broccoli. Tofu set with calcium and calcium-fortified orange juice are also good sources. So don't pay any attention to the latest milk mustaches, or ads implying that milk is necessary for your health. Try soymilk or almond milk to drink, and eat plenty of green leafy vegetables. Your bones will thank you for it.

Will a vegetarian diet help me avoid diabetes or improve my condition if I already have it?

You won't be surprised when we tell you that diet is the main culprit behind diabetes. We've all noticed that as the American diet worsens, the incidence of diabetes gets worse too. Diabetes is a serious disease that is becoming more and more common. Eleven percent of men and 9 percent of women over the age of twenty now have diabetes, and in most cases the cause is diet related. A balanced vegetarian diet goes a long way toward preventing people from getting diabetes, and easing the severity of the disease in those who already have it.

Here's what goes wrong when diabetes strikes. Diabetes is a disease in which the body does not produce or properly utilize insulin, the hormone needed to convert the glucose in the blood into energy in our bodies. Having diabetes means more than just taking insulin or medication. The disease damages the blood vessels and can lead to blindness, kidney and heart disease. It can shave ten to fifteen years off a person's life.

There are two types of diabetes. Type 1 develops when the body cannot produce enough insulin. This often starts in childhood, and there have been several studies showing a strong connection to drinking cow's milk, especially in baby formula. In Finland, the country where they drink the most milk, they have the highest levels of type 1 diabetes, whereas in Japan where they drink very little milk, there are very few cases of type 1 diabetes. Breast-feeding, or using soy-based formula, is the best way to prevent a child from developing this serious disease.

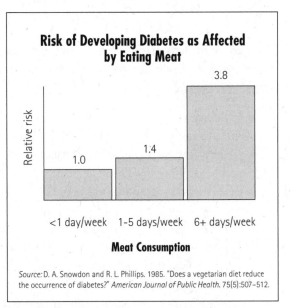

Risk of Developing Diabetes as Affected by Eating Meat

Relative risk

- <1 day/week: 1.0
- 1-5 days/week: 1.4
- 6+ days/week: 3.8

Meat Consumption

Source: D. A. Snowdon and R. L. Phillips. 1985. "Does a vegetarian diet reduce the occurrence of diabetes?" *American Journal of Public Health.* 75(5):507–512.

Figure 2. Meat consumption can increase your risk of developing diabetes.

Type 2 diabetes, where the body fails to properly use the insulin it produces, is much more common than type 1 diabetes. Vegetarians have been found to have only one-quarter the rate of type 2 diabetes, compared with meat eaters. The risk of getting this type of diabetes rises with the more meat you eat in a typical week. But it's not just cutting out the meat that matters. Fruits, vegetables, grains, nuts, and legumes all provide protection against diabetes, so vegetarians tend to be able to use the insulin their bodies make more effectively.

Gregory Scribner, MD, an internist from the state of Washington, says, "A switch to a healthy vegetarian diet can help reverse many of the complications of diabetes, even in advanced cases, and can often prevent the disease from occurring in the first place." If you already have diabetes, it's worth changing your diet as soon as possible. A vegan diet may help to limit complications from the disease, and diabetics who follow a nutritious vegetarian diet for several months may be able to decrease their medication under their doctor's supervision.

My grandfather died of a heart attack. Will a vegetarian diet help prevent me from getting heart disease?

You're right to be worried about getting a heart attack. Heart disease is the most common cause of death in the United States. More than one million people have a heart attack each year, and about half of first heart attacks are fatal which means that the victim doesn't get a second chance.

Heart disease starts young. You may think that heart attacks only happen to older people, so you can wait to change your diet. But plaque, the substance that blocks arteries, starts to accumulate on the artery walls very early in life, and builds up over time. Studies done on American soldiers killed in the Korean and Vietnam Wars showed that at an average age of only twenty-two years, most of them had striking signs of clogged arteries, compared with South Korean and South Vietnamese soldiers who were nearly vegetarian. Another study, published in the American Journal of Medicine, found that 80 to 90 percent of young adults already had substantial amounts of plaque partially clogging their coronary arteries by the time they reached their thirties.

Cholesterol counts. Of all the factors thought to affect heart disease, the amount of cholesterol in your bloodstream (measured as milligrams per deciliter, or mg/dl) is by far the most important. The largest study ever done on the causes of heart disease was carried out in Framingham, Massachusetts. This study found that coronary artery disease, the most common form of heart disease, could be prevented or even reversed in people who kept their cholesterol levels down around 150 mg/dl. This occurred only when the diet followed was a vegetarian one.

The reason for this is simple. Our bodies make all the cholesterol that we need, so there is no need for us to eat any. The cholesterol we eat comes only from animal products—meat, fish, eggs, and dairy foods, including the low or non-fat ones—so when we eat these foods we get all that extra cholesterol included. Unlike animal products, plant foods—including all fruits, legumes, nuts, oils, seeds, and vegetables—contain no cholesterol at all.

Table 1. Cholesterol content of various foods

Animal-based foods	Serving size	Cholesterol content, in milligrams	Plant-based foods	Cholesterol content, in milligrams
egg	1 egg	274	all fruits	0
shrimp	3 ounces	166	all grains	0
pork tenderloin, lean	4 ounces	106	all legumes	0
beef, top round, lean	4 ounces	103	all nuts	0
chicken breast, skinless	4 ounces	97	all seeds	0
salmon, chinook	4 ounces	96	all vegetables	0
turkey breast, skinless	4 ounces	79	all vegetable oils	0
halibut	4 ounces	47		
whole milk	1 cup	34		
swiss cheese	3 ounces	70		
low-fat milk, 2% fat	1 cup	18		
butter	1 tablespoon	11		

Sources: Pennington, Jean, *Bowes and Church's Food Values of Portions Commonly Used*, 16th ed. (Philadelphia: Lippincott, Williams, and Wilkins, 1994); USDA National Nutrient Database.

But there's more to this story. Saturated fats, present in high levels in most animal products, stimulate our livers to produce additional cholesterol, and this is a major factor as well. Take a look at the table showing where saturated fats come from, and compare animal fats to plant fats (called oils because they are not solid at room temperature).

Table 2. Saturated fat in various foods

Animal fats	Saturated fat*
butter	68
beef fat (tallow)	50
pork fat (lard)	33
chicken fat	30

Plant oils	Saturated fat*
olive oil	13
corn oil	13
sunflower oil	10
safflower oil	9
canola oil	7

Sources: Pennington, Jean, *Bowes and Church's Food Values of Portions Commonly Used,* 16th ed. (Philadelphia: Lippincott, William, and Wilkins, 1994); USDA National Nutrient Database.

*Saturated fat is shown as a percentage of total fat.

Extra cholesterol is not needed in our bodies, and so gets deposited on the walls of our arteries, forming a hard substance known as plaque. Over time the plaque builds up, and eventually it clogs up the artery so much that blood can no longer pass through. If that artery leads to the heart (a coronary artery), a heart attack occurs. If it leads to the brain, a stroke occurs.

How Arteries Become Clogged

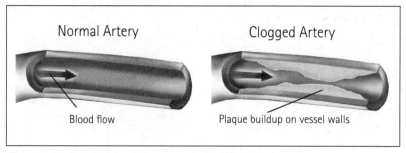

Figure 3. Plaque buildup in arteries can restrict blood flow.

Fruits, vegetables, grains, legumes, and nuts contain no cholesterol and almost no saturated fats, so eating these foods doesn't add to the plaque building up on your artery walls. In fact, if you cut out all animal products from your diet, in a few months the plaque will start to dissolve back into your bloodstream and your arteries will gradually begin to open up.

Texas cardiologist Dean Ornish, MD, discovered this when he took a group of patients who were scheduled for heart bypass operations and put them on a low-fat vegetarian diet. He found that the patients' arteries started to open up, and within a few weeks the patients began to feel improvements. Some of the patients entered this program with severe heart disease. However, within a year, they were able to ride bicycles, play tennis, and even go on long hikes in the Grand Teton Mountains!

This was big news. Although doctors knew vegetarian diets would help prevent heart disease, using a vegetarian diet to reverse heart disease was a major medical advance. Other doctors have since confirmed Ornish's results at several medical centers around the world.

So skip the artery bombs. Frank Hu, MD, professor of nutrition at Harvard School of Public Health, tells it like it is: "Evidence...indicates that a high consumption of plant-based foods, such as fruit and vegetables, nuts, and whole grains, is associated with a significantly lower risk of coronary artery disease and stroke." Cut animal products out of your diet as soon as you can. Your arteries will thank you for it, and you'll have a better chance of living long enough to play with your great-grandchildren.

Can I avoid having a stroke with a vegetarian diet?

You don't want to have a stroke. Stroke is the third leading cause of death in America, and the number one cause of adult disability. A stroke can occur because your blood pressure is too high, causing a blood vessel in your brain to burst, or it can be caused by a blood clot that has formed because an artery has become narrowed due to cholesterol plaque. Either way, a stroke prevents blood, and the oxygen and nutrients it carries, from reaching a part of the brain, and this results in a loss of function. Some people recover completely from a stroke, but more than two-thirds of survivors will have some disability, and some will die. You'll be relieved to know that the risk of having a stroke is significantly reduced when you follow a vegetarian diet.

Besides cigarette smoking, major risk factors for stroke include high blood pressure, high cholesterol, diabetes, obesity, and heart disease. Vegetarians have lower rates of all these diseases, so they also have a lower risk of having a stroke.

In particular, studies have found that vegetarians have one-third to one-quarter the rate of high blood pressure compared to other health-conscious groups of people. Many older people currently take drugs to lower their blood pressure. Studies have found that a change in diet can be just as effective as medication, so if they could just switch to a wholesome vegetarian diet, many would be able to stop the pills, save some money, and get a new lease on life.

Cancer is scary. Can I avoid it by following a vegetarian diet?

Cancer is scary. Many people who get cancer survive thanks to surgery, radiation, and chemotherapy, but cancer is still the second leading cause of death in America, so the most important thing is prevention.

Now for the good news: the risk of getting many forms of cancer can be very significantly reduced by improving your diet. It has been found that up to 60 percent of all cancer is caused by the food we eat. Following a vegan diet can reduce your chances of getting cancer because it eliminates animal products, which are associated with a higher risk of cancer, and contains more plant foods, which are associated with a lower risk.

Don't break the piggy bank! One way that meat, fish, eggs, and dairy products contribute to the risk of cancer is through the toxic environmental chemicals that build up in an animal's flesh over the course of its lifetime, just like money in a piggy bank. Levels of pesticides, such as DDT, and industrial toxic chemicals, such as PCBs and dioxin, are often one hundred times higher in animal products than they are in fruits and vegetables. This is because the animal has eaten pesticide and industrial toxins in its feed throughout its lifetime. Since it is not able to easily eliminate the chemicals it ingests, those chemicals are stored in the flesh of the animal. When we eat that flesh or milk, in the form of meat or dairy products, we receive an animal's lifetime dose of chemicals.

This principle also applies to fish, which eat smaller fish and algae throughout their lives. Many toxic chemicals accumulate in the algae, which become concentrated in the fish higher up the food chain. Freshwater fish, in particular, have been found to have some of the highest levels of industrial toxic chemicals of any food.

In addition to all these toxic chemicals, another group of toxic chemicals, known as heterocyclic amines (HCAs), are formed when meat is cooked. HCAs are known carcinogens, which means that they have been shown to cause cancer. Every meat item, from a burger to a chicken breast, has been found to have high

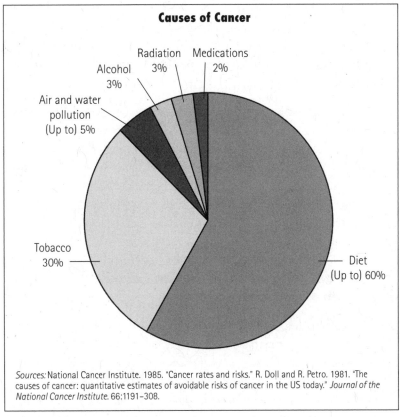

Causes of Cancer

Radiation 3%

Medications 2%

Alcohol 3%

Air and water pollution (Up to) 5%

Tobacco 30%

Diet (Up to) 60%

Sources: National Cancer Institute. 1985. "Cancer rates and risks." R. Doll and R. Petro. 1981. "The causes of cancer: quantitative estimates of avoidable risks of cancer in the US today." *Journal of the National Cancer Institute.* 66:1191–308.

Figure 4. Diet plays a major role in cancer risk.

levels of HCAs after grilling, prompting some health groups to demand that fast-food restaurants label these foods as dangerous to human health. No HCAs are formed when vegetarian products are grilled.

Skip the dogs and the salami. Meat products that have preservatives, such as the nitrates and nitrites found in hot dogs and smoked meats, have also been implicated in several forms of cancer. Some cancer groups now strongly suggest that people avoid processed meat products, such as hot dogs and salami.

Since a vegetarian meal does not contain meat, it avoids all of these problems. In addition, it usually contains more fruits, vegetables, grains, and legumes. There are substances called phytonutrients and antioxidants in plant foods that work to help prevent cancer, so it's no surprise that many studies have shown lower rates of cancer in people consuming a diet high in these foods.

Protect yourself. By not eating meat, fish, eggs, and dairy products, and by eating lots of fruits, vegetables, grains, and legumes, you'll be able to limit your exposure to toxic chemicals, increase the intake of cancer-preventing nutrients, and put the odds of preventing cancer strongly in your favor.

I smoke cigarettes. Can a vegetarian diet help prevent lung cancer?

There's a reason they call cigarettes death sticks. We're sure you know already that smoking cigarettes puts you at risk for many serious diseases including cancer, and that if you can quit smoking you should do so. But what you may not know is that if you cut meat from your diet, and start eating lots of fruits and vegetables, you will be able to reduce your risk of lung cancer by half. While you're trying to give up smoking, replacing meat with lots of fresh fruits and vegetables cuts the risk of not only lung cancer, but cancer in other parts of the body too. This is true for both smokers and non-smokers alike.

I don't want to lose my mind. Can I avoid Alzheimer's disease on a vegetarian diet?

Don't lose your mind for the sake of a cheeseburger. The number of people with Alzheimer's disease is rising rapidly. Alzheimer's disease affects 10 percent of all Americans over 65, and 50 percent of those over age 85. As people succumb to this disease, they start to become forgetful and then lose their ability to think, which is very upsetting for both them and their loved ones. As with many other diseases, a vegetarian diet gives you a very significant health advantage in avoiding Alzheimer's.

Avoid the risk factors. A forty-year study conducted in northern California by Kaiser Permanente found that people with high or even borderline cholesterol had a 66 percent increase in the risk of developing Alzheimer's disease. A study done at Rush University Medical Center in Chicago showed that people with diabetes had up to a 65 percent increased risk. And a third study, carried out by Loma Linda University in California, showed that meat eaters face a 300 percent greater risk of developing Alzheimer's compared to vegetarians. Since following a vegetarian diet lowers your risk of high cholesterol, high blood pressure, and diabetes, it also lowers your risk of Alzheimer's disease. So give yourself the best chance of keeping your brain sharp throughout your life by following a healthful vegetarian diet.

I have flat feet. Will a vegetarian diet help that too?

While it may seem that a vegetarian diet is a prevention or treatment for any problem, there are some health concerns that have nothing to do with your diet. Good nutrition, based on a sound vegetarian diet, can help with healing and repairing your body, and helping it to function the way that it is supposed to, but it can't help fix genetic disorders (although it may help beneficially modify them), soothe sore muscles, heal broken bones, or replace missing teeth and other parts of your body! Nor can it cure the common cold. But a vegetarian diet, and especially a vegan diet, can prevent and reverse the diseases that are the top causes of death, disability, and suffering in the United States—and that's nothing to sneeze at.

CHAPTER 3

For the Animals

Why should I care about farm animals?

Caring is cool. Caring about the lives of innocent and defenseless animals is way cool. We reach our fullest potential as human beings when we start to care about others. Many people feel guilty about having animals killed for their food, especially once they discover that a vegetarian diet can be a tasty and healthful alternative. A lot of people become vegetarians for this reason alone. Killing animals for their meat weighs heavily on their conscience.

Just ask yourself this question: Does it make any sense to care so much for cats and dogs, but to condemn a cow, sheep, or chicken to a life of misery on a factory farm and an early death in a slaughterhouse? Just like cats and dogs, farm animals are sensitive to pain and want to live full, happy lives.

Being killed for food is no fun. There's a saying that if slaughterhouses had glass walls, we'd all be vegetarians. All too often it's "out of sight, out of mind." Most of us don't live near a farm or slaughterhouse, and so we don't witness how harshly the animals are treated. We don't see them being led into the slaughterhouse to be killed for our consumption, we only see the neatly packed cuts of meat in the butcher's shop or grocery store, which no longer look like they were ever a living animal. But that doesn't mean it isn't happening.

Animals are innocent. If they kill, they do so only by instinct. No choice is involved in their actions, but we do have a choice. Many people feel that killing innocent animals violates their sense of justice, and because animals are innocent they deserve our mercy.

The founding fathers spoke out against cruelty to animals. The father of the American Revolution, Thomas Paine, said, "Everything of cruelty to animals is a violation of moral duty." The founder of the state of Pennsylvania, William Penn, said, "It is a cruel folly to offer up to ostentation so many lives of creatures as make up the state of our treats." And Benjamin Franklin, a vegetarian himself, did not mince words when he said, "Flesh eating is unprovoked murder."

Not caring is bad for America. Not caring about animals not only hurts the animals and pains our conscience, but it also damages our society. Indifference to the suffering of animals is a slippery slope that can easily lead to indifference to the suffering of people. It's no secret that many people who commit crimes of cruelty against people, started out by being cruel to animals first.

Some people who care about animals do so for religious reasons. See page 61 for more information.

Do animals feel pain?

If animals can't feel pain, then why do researchers test pain medication on them? Why do they scream or wince when they are hurt? Of course animals feel pain and are capable of suffering. Anthropologist Jane Goodall says, "Farm animals are treated as mere things, yet they are living beings capable of suffering pain and fear." *The Merck Veterinary Manual*, the standard reference in animal science and veterinary practice, states, "Based on what is known to date, all vertebrates, and some invertebrates, experience pain in response to actual or potential tissue damage." In fact, scientists have found pain receptors in mammals, birds, and even fish. If animals could only talk, and therefore beg for their lives, no one except the cruelest person would ever dare kill them. It's time to face the fact that animals do suffer and that they do feel pain.

In our experience, many people try to deny the fact of animal suffering through a complicated and twisted maze of excuses. Some of these excuses come across as nothing less than exercises in denial so that they don't have to change their diet. Another problem is that some people want to claim that the exclusive ability to suffer pain is one of the things that make people exceptional in the animal kingdom. These people are afraid that if they admit that animals can feel pain, too, then humanity has lost one of the things that make us unique. Presidential speechwriter and author, Matthew Scully, responds to this by saying that we should bravely face the fact of animal pain, act more compassionately toward the animals, and "by just and merciful conduct show how exceptional we really are."

Here's the most important question for you to ask yourself. Now that you know that animals suffer pain and fear, what will you do? Isn't making some changes to your diet easier than living with all that pain and misery on your conscience, and having to come up with excuses for every meal?

What exactly is a factory farm?

This isn't going to be easy to read. Factory farms, where most farm animals are raised, treat animals as nothing more than machines in a factory. The animals

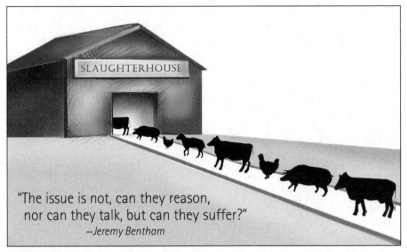

Figure 5. Animals have a right not to suffer.

are run for profit and efficiency of production. Little or no thought is given to their living conditions. The animals are raised in very cramped conditions, fed an unnatural diet, and deprived of everything that would make their lives normal. All too often, undercover videos have been released showing the animals deliberately abused by workers on these farms. Unlike for cats and dogs, there are hardly any laws to protect farm animals, although just recently this has started to change in a small handful of states.

It shouldn't hurt to be a chicken, but it does on factory farms. Chickens have their beaks cut off to prevent them from pecking each other. This is done without any anesthesia. The chickens are then packed into cages so tightly they can't even turn around. There they stay for their whole lives. The cages are stacked on top of one another so their droppings fall onto the chickens below. When eggs are hatched, to provide more egg-laying hens, male chicks are usually not wanted, so they are often thrown into plastic bags and suffocated.

Cows and pigs fare little better. The cows are crowded onto feedlots. Beef calves are taken from their mothers at a young age, branded, dehorned and castrated if male, all without anesthesia, and then kept in a feedlot, where they stand on dirt and their own manure. They are fed an unnatural diet of corn and soy, instead of their natural foods of grass and scrub, and pumped full of antibiotics and hormones (unless they are organic) to make them gain weight faster. Mother pigs (sows) are often kept in gestation pens so small they can't turn around, and their babies have to suckle through the sides of the pen until they are weaned. They can never snuggle up close, and are then crammed into pens with many others until they grow big enough for slaughter. Not surprisingly, factory farmed animals often suffer health problems due to their unnatural diet and dreadful living conditions.

When you choose vegetarian food, based on fruits, vegetables, grains, and legumes, you can feel comfort from the knowledge that no farm animals were harmed in the production of your meal.

What happens in slaughterhouses?

Animals don't want to die, and do their best to avoid being killed. We'll spare you the details of their experiences in the slaughterhouse, but despite the Humane Slaughter Act of 1978 (which doesn't cover chickens and turkeys), you can be sure that many of them are not killed humanely. Videos documenting abuse in slaughterhouses are disturbing beyond description. There's a good reason why slaughterhouses don't have glass walls!

Will consuming eggs and dairy still result in animal suffering?

Those who have cut out meat but still consume eggs and dairy products because the animals are not directly killed, are well intentioned. At one time, it was not that hard on an animal to supply eggs or milk, but with factory farming that is no longer the case. Unfortunately these days, dairy and egg production cause a lot of animal suffering. The objective of a dairy or egg farmer is to produce as much milk or as many eggs as possible for the least possible cost, so farmers give very little thought to caring for the animals, except to ensure that they continue to produce. Dairy cows and egg-laying chickens have miserable lives and end up in the slaughterhouse just like their meat-producing relatives.

In order to keep producing milk, dairy cows are forced to give birth as frequently as possible, but their calves are taken away from them shortly after birth, so that the milk they produce is available for human use. Often they are injected with recombinant bovine growth hormone (rBGH), which is designed to produce an abnormally high volume of milk. Many develop mastitis, a painful infection of the udders, and lameness. When their milk production wanes after about three or four years, they are sent to slaughter.

The baby calves produced in this process are either raised to produce milk themselves, if they are female, or sometimes raised for veal if they are male. These poor animals are deliberately fed a diet that puts them at risk of becoming anemic and kept in small crates to prevent their muscles developing. This creates the kind of pale, soft meat prized as veal.

So the lives of dairy- and egg-producing animals are full of suffering and end in slaughter, in much the same way as those of the meat-producing animals. With so many delicious alternatives available, causing this much pain to animals is just not necessary.

Are organic and free-range farm animals treated better?

I wish we had good news for you but we don't. Some farmers in this category do treat their animals with a bit more compassion, but most do not. With no legal definition of "free range," there is no way to hold the producer accountable. Often free-range animals, while not technically caged, are crammed into sheds so tightly it amounts to almost the same thing. The term "organic" only refers to the feed and the use of antibiotics in a given farm animal, but doesn't say much about its overall living conditions.

With a wide variety of unregulated terms in use, it can be very difficult to determine how an animal was raised, based on the labeling in the grocery store. None of the labels apply to how the animal was transported or slaughtered. Almost all animals raised for food suffer pain during their lives. Still, if you're not ready to give up meat, choosing organic or free-range meat is a step in the right direction, albeit a small one.

Battery-caged Hens

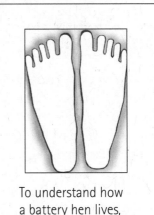

To understand how a battery hen lives, stand here for a year.

Figure 6. Battery hens live their lives in tiny cages.

Do fish have it any better?

Fish suffer too. Individual fish enjoy a normal life until they're caught, but scientists have found that even fish are capable of suffering pain. The fishing industry makes no effort to minimize the trauma fish experience when caught. One in three fish are thrown back into the sea, dead or dying, because they are not the type of fish needed in that catch. The long nets used to catch fish also catch

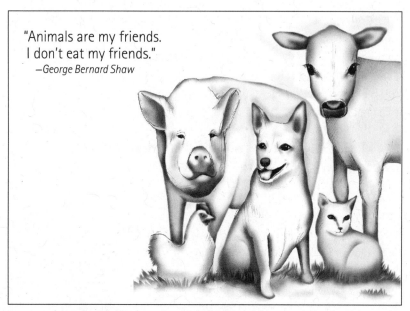

"Animals are my friends.
I don't eat my friends."
—*George Bernard Shaw*

Figure 7. A love for animals means not eating them.

sensitive sea mammals, such as dolphins, porpoises, and seals, which become additional casualties of the fishing industry.

Fish belong in the ocean. Fish farming, however, involves raising fish in huge pens, where they are fed concentrated protein pellets to encourage fast growth. These fish cannot swim freely and suffer from overcrowding. Diseases and parasites, which would normally exist in relatively low levels in fish scattered around the oceans, can run rampant in densely packed fish farms. So fish farms increase the level of suffering experienced by fish.

Don't plants feel pain too?

It's amazing how some people try to bob and weave in order to avoid facing unpleasant facts. If you stress the cruelty to animals as your main reason for going vegetarian, some people are bound to raise the issue of plants, trying to show you that you really can't eat anything if you worry about the impact on what you're eating. Of course the real answer to this is that plants don't have a nervous system or pain receptors, so they can't feel pain. You can point out that animals show that they feel pain by wincing or making a sound (if they can), whereas there is no visible reaction to pain from a plant. The ultimate answer to give these people is that even if plants did feel pain, many more plants had to die to feed the animal to give us meat than if we just ate the plants directly.

I care about animals but I wonder how many others do?

If you care about the animals and value their lives, you're not alone. Caring about animals has never been more popular in America. An opinion poll commissioned by the Associated Press found that two-thirds of Americans believe that an animal has a right to live free of suffering. In addition, one-third of Americans are worried that the existing laws to protect animals are inadequate. That same concern has also been contributing to the rise of mainstream animal welfare organizations. For instance, the Humane Society of the United States now boasts over 11 million members.

If the situation for farm animals is so bad, how come it is allowed to continue?

In order for people to react against animal suffering, they have to know about it first. If the facts are hidden or presented to them in a way they find objectionable, people don't take action.

Part of the problem is that eating meat is a longstanding custom for most people. Because meat eating is an everyday act for many people, they don't think about the extraordinary ethical issues it raises. As British playwright George Bernard Shaw once observed, "Custom will reconcile people to any atrocity." Unfortunately, this is the case with eating meat.

Other people are simply in denial. They know the facts but refuse to face up to them, because facing up to unpleasant facts is psychologically uncomfortable. While going into denial might make some people feel better, that comfort comes at a high price for the animals.

Some people want everything to be OK. Recently, there has been a disturbing trend for some people to regard *everything* as acceptable. While this trend started out with the noble goal of promoting tolerance, it has instead led to the legitimization of some of the most harmful acts in society. All too often in today's society, people are too afraid of political incorrectness to take a stand against what they believe is wrong. But a society that can't recognize some things as wrong can't improve. People who choose a vegetarian diet, because they believe it is wrong to kill an animal after raising it in misery, are saying, in effect, that some things are just not acceptable.

Do some people become vegetarians out of a reverence for life?

Many people see life as precious. Paul McCartney of the Beatles put it well when he said, "We don't eat anything that has to be killed for us. We've been through a lot and we've reached the stage where we really value life." Many people consider a vegetarian diet to be a life-affirming diet. By making vegetarian food choices, you will be saving the lives of many farm animals and, in all probability, saving your own life as well.

CHAPTER 4

For the Environment

How does eating a vegetarian diet help the environment?

Massive is the only word we can think of when it comes to the damage to the environment caused by raising livestock. Since one-third of all the habitable land in the world is used for raising animals (or for growing crops to feed them), it's not surprising that the animal agriculture industry has such a massive impact on our environment. Farm animals require huge amounts of feed, and the fertilizers and pesticides used to grow that feed are made from oil or use it in their production. Raising farm animals takes enormous quantities of fresh water for drinking and for growing their feed, and fossil fuel to power all the equipment, transportation, refrigeration, and freezing that raising meat requires. Livestock produce greenhouse gases, pollute water with their waste, and require ever more land to live on, resulting in ecological destruction.

You can make a big difference through the food choices you make. By choosing to follow a vegetarian diet, you are reducing the demand for meat and other animal products. This in turn has an impact on how many animals farmers decide to raise, how many resources they use, and how much pollution will be caused. While the impact of one person's dietary change may seem small, as more and more people make this choice, the effects really add up. If everyone were to go vegetarian, there would be no need for a meat industry at all, and environmental problems such as global warming, water pollution, and rainforest destruction would be drastically reduced.

Why does animal agriculture use so much oil?

It's amazing how much oil is used to produce meat. In fact, agriculture uses 17 percent of all the fossil fuel (oil, coal, and natural gas) in the United States, with meat production responsible for the majority of that portion. There are several reasons for this. One reason is that most animals are raised in so-called factory farms, where their feed is grown elsewhere and shipped in. These animals consume enormous quantities of crops—in fact about 70 percent of all the corn and 80 percent of all the soybeans grown in the United States are fed to farm animals. When we consider the fossil fuel used for meat production, we also have to take into account all the fuel used to manufacture fertilizers and pesticides, and to water, harvest, and ship those crops throughout the animal's entire lifetime, as well as the fuel required for the transportation and slaughter of the animals, plus the shipping and refrigeration of the meat. All that fuel adds up. Grass-fed animals use less fuel, but these animals use so much land that it's not practical to feed America's meat habit this way.

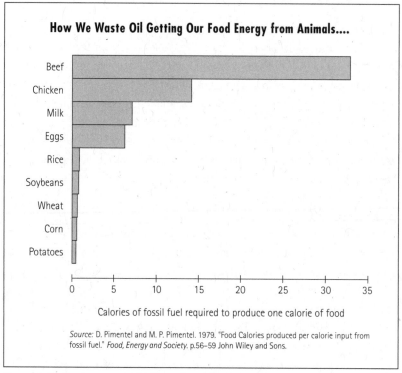

How We Waste Oil Getting Our Food Energy from Animals....

Calories of fossil fuel required to produce one calorie of food

Source: D. Pimentel and M. P. Pimentel. 1979. "Food Calories produced per calorie input from fossil fuel." *Food, Energy and Society.* p.56–59 John Wiley and Sons.

Figure 8. The food we eat greatly affects the world's fuel supply.

Going vegetarian saves oil. Plant-based foods are simply grown, harvested, shipped, and eaten directly rather than wastefully being funneled through a farm animal first. Much less refrigeration is usually required for plant foods than animal products. But the big advantage is that it takes only a pound of grain to make a loaf of bread, whereas it takes more than seventeen pounds of grain to make a pound of beef, requiring much more fossil fuel.

How is global warming affected by eating meat?

Global warming just may be the most serious environmental threat in human history. It's caused by the production of large quantities of greenhouse gases, such as carbon dioxide and methane. These gases trap heat in the earth's atmosphere and so contribute to the overwarming of the planet. Many scientists are very concerned that this warming is causing the glaciers and the polar ice caps to melt, which is causing a gradual rise in sea levels. Low-lying lands are at risk of being permanently flooded, causing many people to lose their homes and farmland. In other parts of the world, changes in weather patterns, cause droughts that in turn cause famine. If the world continues to produce or increase global warming gases at the current rate, there will be an environmental catastrophe that could lead to the death of millions of people.

In the previous question, we saw just how much fossil fuel is consumed in the production of meat, and this of course is a major source of carbon dioxide. But the animals also produce carbon dioxide when they breathe, and many produce huge quantities of methane as flatulence and from their manure. Methane is twenty-one times more effective than carbon dioxide at heating the atmosphere. Since 56 billion farm animals worldwide are raised for food each year (eight times the human population), you can see that, added together, animals produce a huge share of the greenhouse gases that are causing our planet to warm up.

Get ready for this one. According to a report from the United Nations Food and Agriculture Organization, raising livestock causes more global warming than all the cars, buses, trucks, airplanes, boats, and ships in the world put together. It turns out that whether or not you eat meat is much more important than whether or not you have a fuel-efficient car, whether or not you carpool or take public transportation, whether or not you buy local, and whether or not you vacation close to home.

Nothing is more important in the fight against global warming than becoming a vegetarian. By switching to a vegetarian diet, you can single-handedly reduce greenhouse gases by 3,267 pounds per person per year. If enough other people follow your lead, the biggest source of greenhouse gases would be removed, and global warming wouldn't be the impending crisis that it is today.

How does the use of water to produce meat cause problems?

You might think, especially if you live in the Pacific Northwest where it feels like it never stops raining, that water is no big deal. But if you live in a drier place, like California, Arizona, or further afield in parts of Africa, Asia, and Australia, water is a really big deal. People around the globe engage in continual debates, arguments, and even battles over how to share scarce water resources from local rivers and streams. Fresh water is needed for basic human needs like drinking and washing. It's used for industry, agriculture, and in some places for hydro-electric power, and it's used for recreation (fishing, boating) and watering lawns and golf courses. In dry parts of the world, where there is not enough water to go around, major compromises have to be made. Often these compromises work in favor of the people willing to pay the most, and so poorer people lose out on what should be a basic human right: access to clean, fresh water.

Watering crops and grassland to feed farm animals is a huge waste of water. By some estimates, every pound of beef produced requires 5,214 gallons of water to grow the crops that feed the cow and to provide water for the cow to drink. Compare that to wheat or tomatoes or lettuce, which need less than twenty-five gallons of water per pound of food. When countries choose to raise animals for food, rather than feed their people crops directly, they are wasting precious fresh water, which is desperately needed for other uses.

Since meat in Western countries may come from many different sources, it's very difficult to track down where the meat you eat has been raised, and where the crops it was fed were grown. But every time you choose a vegetarian meal, you can be sure that you are saving someone a substantial amount of water, which can be put to a more productive use.

How does raising animals cause ecological destruction?

Raising farm animals and harvesting fish are the biggest causes of ecological destruction on both land and sea. On land, ecological destruction is caused by overgrazing, which leads to soil erosion and desertification, and by the destruction of natural habitats, such as the Amazon Rainforest. In the oceans, industrial fishing causes massive disruption of the food chain and the underwater ecology.

The fires burning in the Amazon are so bright that astronauts can see them from space. Cattle ranchers in Brazil, which is now a major meat-exporting country, set these fires to clear land to raise beef, and to raise crops such as soybeans to feed the cows. In only ten years, an area twice the size of Portugal was burned down mostly just to clear land to raise beef. And in Central America, half the rainforest has already been destroyed in order to raise farm animals. Rainforest destruction is a continuing tragedy. The rainforest is home to many rare plants and animals, which are losing their habitat and are thus at risk for extinction. In addition, once the forest has been cleared, the land is particularly susceptible to soil erosion. David Kaimowitz, director of the Center for International Forestry Research, doesn't pull any punches when he says, "Cattle ranchers are making mincemeat out of Brazil's rainforests."

Fishing is destroying the ocean's ecology. Long nets used by industrial fishing boats catch many nonfood species of fish, which are then thrown back dead or dying. These species, which have been killed for no useful purpose, are removed from the oceanic food chain causing massive ecological destruction. Fish farming also generates a lot of waste. These fish are held in pens and are fed huge amounts of concentrated protein pellets. The leftover pellets, and the waste from the fish themselves, sink to the bottom of the ocean, generating bacteria that consume the oxygen that shellfish and other bottom-dwelling sea creatures need to survive, thus destroying their habitats.

How does raising livestock cause soil erosion?

It's hard to get excited about dirt but our lives depend on it. Food crops can't grow without soil and without the crops we all face starvation. Soil is formed through a natural process of wind and water on the earth, but this is a slow process. For example, in Iowa it takes 200 years to form one inch of topsoil. Plants and vegetation bind the soil together, but when those plants are removed, due to grazing or farming crops to feed animals, there is nothing to stop the soil from being washed or blown away. In Iowa, soil is being removed thirty times faster than it is being formed. Across the country, 85 percent of all soil erosion is due to raising livestock. With 56 billion farm animals raised in the world each year, and one-third of the habitable land being used directly or indirectly to raise them, scientists are sounding the alarm as massive soil erosion continues unabated. In parts of the United States, China, and sub-Saharan Africa, soil erosion has turned what was once valuable farming land into desert.

How does raising animals pollute the water and the air?

Nobody wants dirty water and smelly air. Some of the most obnoxious environmental damage caused by raising animals is due to the waste they produce. Cows and pigs in particular, but even chickens, produce enormous quantities of waste. In fact, here in the United States, farm animals produce over 130 times more poop than the human population. Some can be used as fertilizer but most of it is stored in piles or lagoons, which can give way. Look out when it rains!

Most of it winds up either seeping into the groundwater or running into the lakes and streams, causing pollution in these bodies of water and massive fish kills in the process. The groundwater surrounding these farms often has nitrate levels far above government standards because of all the seepage from animal waste. Increased nitrate levels have been linked to an increased risk of both cancer and miscarriage.

What a stink! The smell from all this waste is indescribable. Even people living some distance away are affected. Just imagine having to live with that smell day in and day out. The smell is often so intense that even helicopters and small planes flying overhead get treated to the stink.

What can I do about it?

The power to protect the environment is in your hands. Animal agriculture, and the crops needed to feed them, is a huge industry that causes untold damage to our environment. Every time you choose a vegetarian meal instead of a meat-based one, you are helping to limit that damage and taking a powerful step toward a more sustainable world.

CHAPTER 5

For the World's Hungry

How bad is the global hunger crisis?

Starvation hurts. Hunger and malnutrition are some of the most serious problems facing humanity and it's getting worse. Global hunger is at an all-time high, with about 1 billion people in the world going to bed each night hungry. In the next year, more than 10 million people will actually starve to death. Unfortunately, it's the children who are the most vulnerable.

Why should I care about the hungry?

What do you do when you get hungry—reach for something in the kitchen, grab a bite from the fridge and throw it in the microwave, or just go out and get something? But what if the kitchen was empty, or there was no fridge and nowhere to go out to? What would you do then?

This is the position a large number of people find themselves in every day. They either have no food or they don't have enough to get by, so they go to bed hungry day after day. For many, it means nothing less than a slow death. Now put yourself in their shoes and imagine how it feels to starve. If you've ever skipped a few meals you know what it's like to feel hungry and weak. Just imagine spending the rest of your life that way.

Responsibility is not a dirty word. The hungry of the world are your brothers and sisters, and we all have a responsibility to care about them and care for them. Don't give in to "out of sight, out of mind." Just because the hungry are out of your everyday sight doesn't mean they should be out of your mind.

Now think with your heart. After all, it's your heart more than anything else that makes you human. Your heart will tell you that caring is the right thing to do.

Why is global hunger increasing?

There are two reasons for the worsening levels of hunger. One is that the world's population continues to increase. It's now at almost 7 billion, and predicted to be over 9 billion by 2050.

Here's the part most people don't know about. An even bigger factor in world hunger, which is not so often discussed, is that more and more developing countries—China in particular—are greatly increasing the amount of meat they consume. As they raise more meat, they need more grain to feed the animals, and so they start to import grain, whereas previously they were self-sufficient.

Hey Buddy, can you spare a few million tons of wheat? What does a country do when they don't have enough grain of their own? They import it. For instance, once the leading producer of soybeans in the world, China is now the leading importer, mostly from the United States. China will need to import 300 million tons of grain by the year 2020 if it continues to turn toward a meat-based diet.

China isn't the only country in this situation. Ethiopia, Nigeria, Iran, Pakistan, and Indonesia are among a host of other nations that have become net importers of grain, fueled mostly by the growth of their livestock sectors. By the year 2030, Bangladesh and Ethiopia are expected to increase their grain imports by a factor of nine, Indonesia and Iran by a factor of four.

There's a world of waste in the current system of taking our crops and feeding them to farm animals. Globally, 90 percent of the soybean harvest and 40 percent of the grain is now used for animal feed. And, as you'll see in the next section, most of the nutrition is wasted by the animals and never appears in the form of meat. This enormous waste is driving hunger and malnutrition in the hungry regions of the world.

How can following a vegetarian diet help the hungry people of the world?

Let's start with the agricultural facts of life. Farm animals function, in effect, as food factories in reverse; that is, they give us less nutrition than they are fed. For instance, a cow will give us as beef only 10 percent of the protein and 4 percent of the calories it consumes. The rest is used by the cow to enable it to live and breathe throughout its lifetime. With 56 billion farm animals raised globally each year, you can see just how much food is being wasted. Wasting food by feeding it to farm animals fuels the global hunger crisis. With developing countries quickly changing from their traditional plant-centered diet to a Western-style, meat-centered diet, it's easy to see how hunger and malnutrition can spread. Many of these people live in countries that could feed themselves, but farmers, policy makers, and governments choose to feed crops to farm animals instead of people. The result is that they often need to import grain to feed their human population. This is expensive and drives up prices. A rising global population makes wasting food this way even more harmful.

How We Waste Protein and Calories

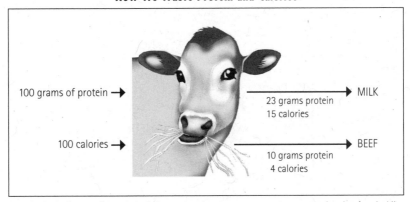

100 grams of protein →

100 calories →

→ MILK
23 grams protein
15 calories

→ BEEF
10 grams protein
4 calories

Figure 9. Only a small amount of the energy that cows consume is converted to beef and milk.

Raising meat is just plain crazy. Growing crops to feed farm animals not only replaces inexpensive nutritional protein with expensive nutrition, but also reduces the total amount available for human consumption because so much is wasted by the animal.

Vegetarian diets are the solution to global hunger or, at the very least, the biggest part of it. With few exceptions, those countries with chronic hunger and malnutrition problems could feed themselves if they would only take the crops they feed to animals and make them available for people instead. These countries would also save a lot of money since they would no longer need to pay for imported food.

Yes, the world's population is rising quickly, and that puts pressure on global food supplies, but a vegetarian diet could easily support a world population much larger than today's. With a rising population, the only sustainable way out of the global hunger crisis is by reducing meat consumption or becoming vegetarians.

Why can't we just grow more food?

Not all acres are created equal, and good new farmland is getting harder and harder to find. The world is running out of quality farmland. Many people think that there is plenty of farmland around the world just waiting to be cultivated. This is not the case. With the notable exception of the United States, almost all of the world's prime farmland is already being used. The remaining farmland is of very poor quality, and it doesn't produce food efficiently. Thomas Homer-Dixon, a professor in the faculty of environment at the University of Waterloo,

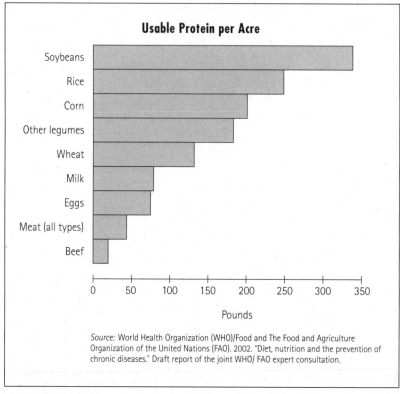

Figure 10. Plant foods produce more protein per acre when eaten directly than when converted into meat.

explains, "Nearly all the best farmland is already being used. Most of what's left is either less fertile, not sufficiently rainfed or easily irrigated, infested with pests, or harder to clear, plant, and plow."

Raising animals for food is a monumental waste of land. Figure 10 shows that an acre of land will yield 356 pounds of protein if it is used to grow soybeans, but only twenty pounds if it is used to raise beef. Seventeen times more protein can be obtained by eating plants directly rather than by first feeding them to animals and then eating the plants "secondhand." The most efficient use of that land is raising food for people, not animals.

The environment takes a hit from using marginal farmland. In many parts of the world, especially in rainforest regions such as the Amazon, people are cutting down forests to clear land for animal grazing. In addition to the loss of habitat for wild plants and animals, and the loss of the trees to absorb carbon dioxide from the atmosphere, this also causes a big problem with soil erosion. Once the trees are gone, the soil is no longer bound into the tree roots, and so it is easily washed away by rains or blown away by the wind. The loss of topsoil makes the land less fertile and it doesn't take long for such land to become unable to produce the crops or grasslands for which it was cleared in the first place. In some places it even becomes a desert. As the world's deserts increase, due to both overgrazing and global warming, less and less land is available for farming. What the world needs is to make better use of the farmland already in use.

The oceans are huge, so why don't we feed people more fish?

Nice idea, but it won't work. The world's fisheries are already producing more fish than is sustainable. Eleven of the world's fifteen most important fishing grounds are in decline, and 60 percent of the major fish species are overexploited. If this continues, by the year 2049 there will be no edible species of fish left.

Nearly one in three fish caught are thrown back into the sea, dead or dying each year, because of wasteful fishing practices. One of every three fish caught goes to feed animals, not human beings. Only about one of every three fish harvested from the world's oceans actually goes to feed people. If we were able to ban farmers from feeding fish to animals, there would be more fish available for people, but as the population increases, there still wouldn't be enough.

Aren't war and other catastrophes the real cause of food shortages?

Don't get distracted from the agricultural facts of life. Natural catastrophes, such as earthquakes and floods, grab headlines, and are a factor in food shortages. Warfare and political instability grab attention and can decrease the food supply. But it's the daily waste of food by feeding it to farm animals that's driving the massive global hunger and malnutrition problem. Sure, food is wasted in other ways and sure, there's poverty. But food has always been wasted, and there's always been poverty, yet global hunger is getting worse. What has changed is that meat consumption is skyrocketing in the developing world, which is using up crops that could be used for human consumption.

I thought that some countries were so poor, they could never feed their people. Isn't this the real cause of their hunger?

Poverty matters, but raising meat matters more when it comes to global hunger. You may think that the poor countries of the world can't feed themselves, and so require very large amounts of outside assistance. The fact is that, with few exceptions, even the poorest countries could feed themselves without any international aid, if they would only just stop wasting their crops by feeding them to animals. For every meat meal produced, twelve well-balanced vegetarian meals could be produced. But as demand for meat increases, farmers or governments choose to divert more crops to feeding animals, leaving almost none for the people themselves.

How can Americans make a difference?

It may seem that one person can't make much difference, but one person eats three meals a day, 365 days of the year, which adds up to more than a thousand meals. The grain saved by forgoing a thousand meat-based meals could be used to produce 12,000 well-balanced vegetarian meals, so you can see how it adds up pretty quickly. In fact, says David Pimentel, professor of ecology at Cornell University, "If Americans alone took the food currently fed to farm animals in the United States, we would have enough food to feed the entirety of the world's hungry, and we could do it without plowing even one extra acre of farmland." Adopting a vegetarian diet of fruits, vegetables, grains, nuts, and legumes is not only good for you, it is also an act of charity for those who need it the most.

It's a sin to waste food. Aid agencies should designate all food sent to regions of hunger for human consumption only. These meat-free zones, after some readjustment, would soon enable the people there to live in hunger-free zones. Supporting the aid agencies that already have adopted such policies will make a big difference. Examples of such organizations are Vegfam, International Fund for Africa, and Food For Life Global.

CHAPTER 6

For the Spirit

Why is the spiritual aspect of vegetarianism important?

Healthy people need to combine the various things they think and do into a complete whole. Since some sort of spiritual or philosophical orientation is an important part of life for the vast majority of Americans, and often becomes more so as we get older, many people interested in following a vegetarian diet will want to see how it fits in with the rest of their life. Often people find the spiritual reasons for becoming vegetarian very motivating, and find that their decision to become a vegetarian is more sustainable when they fully understand these reasons.

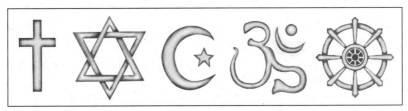

Figure 11. Vegetarianism is compatible with all religions.

Can you give me some examples of vegetarian religious leaders and groups in history?

Thanks be to God, since I gave up flesh and wine I have been delivered from all physical ills.

—**John Wesley**, founder of Methodism

Many famous biblical figures, including Adam, Eve, and Daniel, were vegetarians. The Roman Catholic Church has four vegetarian orders. The Franciscan, Trappist, Benedictine, and Carthusian orders all espouse a vegetarian diet. The founder of Methodism, John Wesley, was a vegetarian, as was the founder of the Salvation Army, General William Booth. Ellen G. White, a founder of the Seventh-day

Adventist Church was a devoted vegetarian. The famous theologian Albert Schweitzer was a vegetarian, too. Martin Luther King's wife, Coretta Scott King, was a vegan, as is his son Dexter Scott King.

Veganism has given me a higher level of awareness and spirituality.

—**Dexter Scott King**, son of Martin Luther King

The first chief rabbi of Israel, Abraham Kook, was a vegetarian. So was chief rabbi Shlomo Goren. The chief rabbi of Haifa is also a vegetarian, as are other important rabbis.

Examples in Eastern religions include the famous Hindu leader, Mahatma Gandhi, and the founder of Buddhism, Gautama Buddha. While we're on the subject of Eastern religion and thought, did you know that Confucius was a vegetarian? In the Muslim world, many people in a sect known as the Sufis also follow a vegetarian diet.

How important to spiritual practice and values is following a vegetarian diet?

Vegetarian diets form an important part of the spiritual practice and values of many people in many religions. How your diet fits into your religion depends on which religious or spiritual orientation you have. While there is plenty of overlap among various religions, each religion has some unique features with regard to food in general and vegetarianism in particular. The food you choose is only one facet of your spiritual life, which may include many other aspects as well, such as faith, prayer, proper behavior, and charity. What you eat should be kept in perspective as part of a greater whole.

How does following a vegetarian diet express Christian values?

The Christian values of reverence for human life, honoring creation, loving your neighbor, and compassion are powerfully expressed by the vegetarian, who preserves human health, sustains the environment, makes more food available to the hungry, and shows compassion to animals. While Christianity does not require a vegetarian diet, more and more Christians are going beyond the minimum requirements and consider a vegetarian diet as a further expression of Christian values in their daily life. In his letter to Philemon, Paul teaches the faithful to do good by voluntarily going beyond the legal minimums, "So that the good [we] do might not be forced but voluntary." (Philem. 14) A vegetarian diet reflects the goodness of Christian values that you achieve when you go the extra mile.

How does following a vegetarian diet express Jewish values?

The Jewish values of preserving life and health, avoiding causing pain to animals, preserving natural resources, and providing food for the poor are all embodied in a vegetarian diet. In fact, the Talmud says that "man ideally should not eat meat." Given the harsh conditions on factory farms and what we know about the effect of meat on our health, global hunger, and the environment, some rabbis have begun to say that meat is no longer acceptable under Jewish law. While some meat technically may be kosher, it still violates other Jewish laws.

Many rabbis also point out that the Torah states that the original diet meant for mankind was vegetarian, and that the prophets teach that the diet in the world to come will again become vegetarian. Also, the book of Daniel describes, in a very compelling way, how greater health is obtained by following a vegetarian diet. Finally, nowhere in the Torah is there a commandment to eat meat.

What Buddhist values are expressed by following a vegetarian diet?

Four of the major themes that run throughout Buddhism are the importance of great wisdom and great compassion, the interconnectedness of all living beings, and the importance of generating good *karma* (the law of how good and bad actions affect the future). The vegetarian diet expresses these values well; it is a very wise diet, because it is good for our health and the health of the environment, it is compassionate, it honors our interconnectedness with the animals, and it does not result in bad *karma* since it does not harm other conscious beings (humans or animals).

Buddha's admonition not to eat meat couldn't be clearer when he says, "Whoever consumes meat extinguishes the seed of great compassion." The Dalai Lama advocates a vegetarian diet, saying, "I do not see any reason why animals should be slaughtered to serve as human diet when there are so many substitutes. After all, man can live without meat."

What Hindu values are expressed by following a vegetarian diet?

Two fundamental concepts of the Hindu scripture are *ahimsa* (the practice of not causing harm to other living beings) and *karma*.

In the Vedic scriptures there are many passages that support vegetarianism. One passage states, "Having well considered the origin of flesh foods, and the cruelty of fettering and slaying corporeal beings, let man entirely abstain eating flesh." Emphasizing the Hindu concept of the unity of all life, Srila Prabhupada, the founder of the Hare Krishna movement, said, "Everyone is God's creature, although in different bodies and dresses."

Perhaps one of the most famous vegetarians of recent times is Mahatma Gandhi, who said, "I do feel that spiritual progress does demand at some stage that we should cease to kill our fellow creatures."

What Muslim values are expressed by following a vegetarian diet?

Mohammed was thought to be concerned about the welfare of animals. The Koran says, "There is not an animal on the earth, nor a flying creature flying on two wings, but they are peoples like unto you." Tradition, or *hadith*, quotes Mohammed as saying, "Whoever is kind to the lesser creatures of God is kind to himself." With this in mind, a Muslim would have a definite basis for selecting a vegetarian diet.

However, except for a mystical Muslim sect called Sufis, and the Hunza, a group that lives in the foothills of the Himalayas in northern Pakistan, vegetarianism has not been widespread among Muslims. This may be beginning to change as some Muslims are starting to explore the benefits of a vegetarian diet. It should be mentioned that the Hunza are acknowledged to be the healthiest people in the entire world.

Are there some other smaller religions that also advocate a vegetarian diet for their followers?

In the Sikh religion, originating in India, the Namdhari sect and the Bhajan Golden Temple movement are strictly vegetarian. According to Sikh scholar Swaran Singh Sanehi, "Sikh scriptures support vegetarianism fully." The Jain religion, also originating in India, follows the *ahimsa* principle (not causing harm to other living beings) quite strictly. The Jains are famous for their devotion to and advocacy of vegetarianism.

Have there been great thinkers and philosophers who taught the vegetarian way?

Some of the biggest names in philosophy have spoken out against using animals for food. While these philosophers were all people of deep faith, often their support of vegetarianism was advocated in a secular context as well as a religious one.

The concerns of the great philosophers who supported the vegetarian way were mostly centered on the harsh treatment of animals raised for food, and how such treatment would affect mankind. For instance, the German philosopher Immanuel Kant warned that hardening our hearts toward animals would affect our dealings with other humans. Voltaire, a well-known French philosopher, took issue with some people of his day who had no regard for animals at all, saying, "How pitiful and what poverty of mind, to have said that animals are machines deprived of understanding and feeling." Another French philosopher, Rousseau, thought that eating meat was not part of the natural human diet.

The famous Roman philosopher, Seneca, and the great Greek philosophers Plato, Socrates, and Pythagoras are all thought to have been vegetarians. In fact, until the Renaissance, vegetarians were known as Pythagoreans. Confucius, the famous Chinese ethical philosopher and teacher, was also a vegetarian. These men were all concerned with the cruelty to animals that comes with using them for food.

Nature has endowed man with a noble and excellent principle of compassion, which extends itself also to dumb animals—whence this compassion has some resemblance to a prince towards his subjects. And it is certain that the noblest of souls are the most extensively compassionate.

—**Francis Bacon**, developer of the scientific method

CHAPTER 7

Why Society Isn't Talking About This

Why is it important for America to change the food it eats?

Raising meat is weakening America and threatening our future. That burger at McDonald's may cost only a dollar but it's really very expensive. Meat is costing us dearly in human terms, in terms of health-care costs, and in terms of the quality of our land, air, and waterways.

A country is only as strong as its people are healthy. Meat has cost more American lives than all the wars in history put together. There's a nutritional crisis in America today threatening the health of its people. Deadly diseases such as heart disease, stroke, and some cancers linked to a meat-centered diet are running rampant, causing needless suffering, shortened lives, and a staggering medical bill that our country no longer has the money to pay.

Part of the richness of America comes from our beautiful and bountiful land and waters. Raising the grain needed to feed livestock erodes our soil, the waste produced by livestock pollutes our waters, and the greenhouse gases the animals emit contribute to global warming. Fixing the damage caused by the livestock industry is costing America a fortune.

While America still faces serious threats from abroad, there's also a battle to be fought on the home front. Meat threatens our lives and our land. Seen from this perspective, there are few acts more patriotic than becoming a vegetarian. America has always risen to meet every challenge. A country strong enough to save the world from both fascism and communism can save itself from damaging food choices.

So why isn't society talking about the need to go vegetarian?

It's hard to see a problem when it surrounds you. Meat is everywhere and has become an accepted part of society, so many people simply do not question it.

Eating meat is part of our cultural heritage and, just like our genes, we inherit our culture. Unlike our genes, our culture is something we can change, but that takes time and effort. For culture to change, people first need to see the necessity for that change. With the compelling advantages for a vegetarian diet largely kept out of the popular mind, that change becomes harder to accomplish.

To make matters worse, the vegetarian portion of our cultural heritage has been swept under the rug. The biographies of many famous people leave out the part about their being a vegetarian. This is especially true in books used in schools.

Let's talk business. Meat is big business, very big business. Few people have the courage to challenge it. The meat industry is very savvy when it comes to public relations. They advertise relentlessly, putting their profits ahead of your health in the process. To hide their sins, they make a big deal over charitable contributions to hospitals and breast cancer research for example, while hiding their role in causing many diseases.

Politicians of both parties refrain from challenging the meat industry for fear of losing campaign contributions. They also know that most people eat meat, so they fear losing votes if they tell people something they don't want to hear. A misplaced and perverted sense of political correctness drives fear into the minds of many policymakers and administrators when it comes to the problem of meat. Often these people have a mindset that insists that every lifestyle choice is acceptable, including meat-centered diets that lead to an early death and environmental degradation, so they avoid dealing with the issue.

Ducking food issues is common in most of society's other institutions as well. For instance, most doctors ignore the results of medical research, and the educational establishment is in denial when it comes to the massive damage caused by producing and consuming animal products.

Why is it so hard for some people to face the facts about food?

Food can be a very emotional issue. One reason some people want to avoid or deny the facts about eating animal products is that they have an emotional connection to eating meat. They may enjoy the flavor and texture of meat, they may associate eating meat with being wealthy or strong, or they may have strong family memories of eating meat and feel that it represents their parents' love. Whatever the reason, they don't want to feel obliged to change what they currently eat.

Food has an important social context, so people worry what others will think if they become a vegetarian. Some people want to protect themselves from social disapproval. For others it's a question of money. Fast-food restaurants have emerged as the most inexpensive way to feed a family. What costs less than the dollar menu at McDonalds? Many people simply don't want to hear about spending more money on food. Of course, once the health and environmental costs are taken into account, nothing could be more expensive. Most of the people who eat at fast-food restaurants just don't realize the price they will pay further down the line.

Life is hard. Many people just can't handle another thing to worry about. All they want to do is just get through the day and not think about tomorrow. Change itself takes time and effort, and it's easier to keep on eating the way they always have. Short-term thinking takes over.

Ignorance is bliss. Since so much of the information showing the damage that animal products cause, and the advantages of the vegetarian way, is being hidden from the general public, food issues occupy a low priority in most people's minds. Lack of good information is a critical issue because it allows food myths to persist. Can you believe that it's the twenty-first century and some people still believe you need to eat meat to be healthy?

We all deserve to be treated with respect. When you decide to become a vegetarian, you will sometimes come across people who aren't comfortable listening to the facts about food, for whatever reason. It is best to respect their feelings and not try to force them to listen, or to discuss the facts, if they don't wish to. It's important to be able to disagree without being disagreeable. You can just say that you respect their right to choose the food they eat, and you hope that they will similarly respect your decision to be vegetarian.

Some people say it's all just a matter of opinion. How can we be sure of the facts about food?

We're not asking you to just take our word for it when it comes to the facts about food. There are plenty of facts about food that you can observe for yourself. For example, a trip to a local hospital could show you people who are suffering from disease and death caused by a poor diet. You can visit a factory farm and see for yourself the pollution it causes. You can see the harsh living conditions that the animals are forced to endure.

However, most of us rely on facts that have been found to be true through numerous carefully conducted scientific studies. Once we have a number of studies showing the same result, we can be reasonably sure of the facts. Analysis of the results gives us an accurate picture of the true situation.

Sometimes, when the facts contradict a person's personal preferences or politics, he or she may be tempted to claim that a fact is only an opinion. This is a clever trick. Don't fall for it. There's a big difference between facts and opinions. When someone says to you that the earth is round, or that the sun rises in the east and sets in the west, they aren't just giving you their opinion. They're telling you a fact that can easily be demonstrated to be true. While everyone is entitled to their own opinions, no one is entitled to their own facts.

Another way of evading facts is to subject them to political rather than scientific verification. Just because the majority of people might vote to say that eating meat is good, because they've always eaten that way, that doesn't mean it's necessarily true. While voting may be a fine way to settle political issues, it's a poor way to settle scientific ones.

While science isn't perfect, it's a very powerful tool to help determine the facts, which we ignore at our peril when it comes to nutrition. The facts have been determined with enough certainty to show that a vegetarian diet is healthier for us, and better for the environment and the animals.

Why do some people say there are no bad foods, only different ones?

Many people are operating in the land of make-believe when it comes to facing the realities of our food, how it affects our health and how it came to be on our dinner plate. Instead of facing the facts they construct a fantasy, which goes something like this: Every food is just as good as every other. We can eat anything we want, and there are never any consequences to our health, to the environment, or to the animals, who were only too happy to live a miserable life on a factory farm and then die in a slaughterhouse to feed us. Everything is OK. All foods are equal. All diets are equal.

In the rush to apply a perverted form of political correctness to the science of nutrition, many people, including some dietitians, have chosen to play this game and tell their patients that there are no bad foods, only different ones. After all, wouldn't saying anything else be judgmental?

But just ask yourself this question: If meat, which damages our health and shortens our life when eaten, pollutes the waterways, ruins the rainforests, causes global warming, and requires the killing of innocent animals to produce, isn't bad then what is? Isn't the right to make judgments, in the interests of ourselves and our society, what living in a democracy is all about?

Be sure to tell it like it is. Sometimes a misguided sense of political correctness can get in the way of seeing things as they really are. While it's important to be tolerant and respectful, it's also important not to lose sight of the truth in the process. Science has shown us that some foods promote disease, while other foods promote health. It's much more important to save our health and our environment than to worry about misplaced concerns of political correctness.

Why hasn't my doctor told me to change my diet?

Perhaps the biggest failure of medicine in the past one hundred years or so is not acting on the overwhelming amount of research linking diet with disease. The top three killers of Americans—heart disease, cancer, and stroke—are all strongly linked with the consumption of meat and other animal products. The same goes for other chronic diseases, such as diabetes and high blood pressure. To some extent we're in the same place with meat that we were in with cigarette smoking years ago. The researchers cried out but most doctors didn't listen.

To make matters worse, doctors receive very little training in nutrition. One can only wonder what medical school administrators must be thinking. They are depriving their students of the most effective prevention and treatment strategies to the most common and deadly diseases in America today. But the problem doesn't stop in medical school.

Doctors need to get real. There's a certain blindness in medicine called "technological fundamentalism." Technological fundamentalism in medicine looks to technology as the answer for *all* medical problems. A bad diet is the primary cause of the increase in the common diseases afflicting our society. Instead of facing this, the medical establishment spends an enormous amount of time, energy, and money looking for another drug or gadget to cure such diseases. Technology does have its place, but what America needs the most is better nutrition, not another drug.

Why don't the environmentalists talk about this?

Who's afraid of tofu and veggies? Most environmentalists, that's who! With a very few notable exceptions, the environmental movement has swept the fantastic amounts of environmental damage caused by livestock agriculture right under the rug.

Talk about not seeing the forest for the trees! Livestock agriculture is the number one cause of global warming, the number one cause of ecological destruction on both land and sea, the number one cause of soil erosion, and one of the largest causes of water pollution. Yet looking through environmental science textbooks, you'll find barely a mention of any of these facts.

There's a big disconnect going on in the environmental movement when it comes to agriculture and food. If you've seen the movie *An Inconvenient Truth*, you'll have noticed this phenomenon for yourself. Meat eating was just a little too "inconvenient" for Al Gore to include in his movie, despite being the single largest cause of global warming. The environmental movement makes a point of telling the rest of us to wake up and face the facts, yet as a whole, they seem unwilling to take their own advice.

Fear won't work in the long run. Most environmental groups are afraid of losing members by telling them about the connection between livestock and pollution. But, with every new report documenting the major role livestock agriculture plays in harming the environment, a growing number of their members are beginning to ask them, "Just what are you afraid of?"

Why do aid agencies help people raise farm animals?

It's hard to understand why aid agencies don't encourage vegetarian diets. The math works against feeding crops to animals because only a small percentage of the nutritional value is returned as meat.

The fact is the majority of farm animals are fed crops that could be fed to humans. It takes twelve pounds of food to produce one pound of meat. This is a significant waste of food. As countries encourage the raising of farm animals for meat, they end up importing grain to feed their people. They could easily grow enough food to feed themselves if they didn't feed it to animals.

Many people want to be just like us. People in developing nations often aspire to live a Western lifestyle. They see fast-food restaurants opening up in their cities, and they long to be able to join in the fun. But they don't consider what this lifestyle will cost them in terms of their health, depletion of natural resources, pollution, and animal suffering. Aid agencies try to help them achieve their goals, without considering whether those goals will help the population become well nourished and healthy.

Why don't teachers talk about all the problems associated with meat, fish, dairy, and eggs?

You don't learn everything there is to know in school. Nowhere is this truer than in nutrition. The issue of meat, and all the problems caused by raising and consuming it, may just be the largest blind spot in American education today.

"Don't rock the boat" seems to be an overriding philosophy of many schools. Today's schools and colleges are often more interested in avoiding friction between different groups than in giving students all the facts, and they worry that food issues will become divisive. So they try to avoid bringing attention to the issues and facts about meat and other animal products. Of course their students will pay a very high price for this omission in the long run.

Teachers have some learning to do too. Most teachers, like many other people, have received very little training in nutrition themselves, so they may rely on general knowledge that could be out-of-date or inaccurate. The meat and dairy industries know this, and so they provide educational materials on nutrition to schools free of charge. Of course, you can be sure that those materials imply that meat and dairy products are wholesome foods. Nutrition in general occupies a low priority in most school curricula, so teachers may not find the time to check out the latest information.

Money talks! Schools and colleges, as with many public institutions, are not immune from the influence of politics and money. School lunches, for example, include large quantities of meat, dairy, and eggs because the government encourages farmers to provide these surplus foods to schools very cheaply.

It's popular to gripe about teachers and schools. Teachers and school administrators point out that teaching classes and running schools is much harder than it looks and that support from parents and the community is often lacking. Yes, there's plenty of blame to go around. However, by choosing not to teach students about the advantages of a vegetarian diet, the schools are depriving their students of one of the most valuable lessons they could learn. This lesson would not only extend the lives of their students, but it would also benefit the environment they live in, as well as those suffering from hunger and malnutrition in other countries.

Sorry, but this is one fish we can't let off the hook. We're going to give the schools an F for failing their students where they need help the most. In the long run, meat and other animal foods will claim way more lives and cause much more human suffering than drugs, alcohol, cigarette smoking, AIDS, and war combined. OK, can we get vegetarian issues on the curriculum now?

Why doesn't my religious leader talk much about vegetarianism?

The issue of meat eating is just not on the radar screens of many religious institutions. However, once they become aware of the moral problems surrounding modern-day factory farming, and all the consequences of meat eating, many clergy are more than willing to take up the issue. This is already beginning to happen. Alvin van Pelt Hart, a Christian theologian and Episcopal priest, puts that matter well for all faiths when he says, "We now have scientific evidence that vegetarianism is good for the body. The greatest spiritual teachers have always known that it is good for the soul."

Most often, the subject of vegetarianism gets very little attention in the seminaries where clergymen are trained. This is very similar to the situation in medical schools where nutrition gets very little space in doctors' education. Fortunately this is starting to change for both clergyman and doctors. In the meantime, you may have to share a little of what you have learned in this book, and refer your minister to the books and websites listed in the Resources section (page 167).

Respect is key. More and more these days, congregants are looking to their religious institutions to lead the way on contemporary issues. Fortunately, many religious leaders understand that although the Bible gives people permission to eat meat, it doesn't require them to eat meat or even state that eating meat is desirable. If you would like your religious leader to take up the issue of meat eating, it's important to ask respectfully. Remember, members of the clergy are still learning too, and those who disagree with us still deserve our respect.

What will it take for society to become more open to vegetarianism?

There are positive signs that vegetarianism is becoming more mainstream. You can find veggie burgers and soymilk in most supermarkets these days. Vegetarian cookbooks are now available in almost all bookstores and libraries, and vegetarian options are springing up in restaurants all over the country. Movie stars and sports personalities regularly announce that they've gone veggie. A public health awareness program called Meatless Monday encourages restaurants, school districts, even whole cities, to start each week with vegetarian meals. Change is coming, but slowly.

The more people change their diets, tell their friends and family, and demand more vegetarian options in restaurants and stores, the more it becomes socially acceptable to be vegetarian. The more doctors see that vegetarians are living longer and healthier lives, and see the evidence of scientific studies proving that it works, the more they will gain confidence to recommend a vegetarian diet as a strategy for healing. The more environmentalists see that it is socially acceptable, the more they will feel confident to recommend a vegetarian diet as a way to help heal the world. The more aid agencies see that feeding food to animals in a hungry world is wasting resources, the more they will encourage people to raise crops with which to feed themselves, instead of animals. And the more ministers become aware of the ethical impact of eating meat, the more they will start to consider suggesting vegetarianism to their congregations.

It's up to you. It's up to us. Vegetarians, individually and in organizations across the country, have our work cut out for us. Several tasks fall on our shoulders if we expect to see further meaningful change. We have to represent ourselves more effectively in the marketplace of ideas. Some vegetarian groups haven't always been as responsible as we'd like to see. Remember, people are looking for help, not a hard time, when it comes to their food choices. Yelling at people and calling them names won't help. A friendly and respectful dialogue with the meat-eating world is what the vegetarian movement so badly needs.

Become an ambassador to the meat-eating world. Remember to be diplomatic when representing the vegetarian community, because all of us may be judged by what you say and do. The tools of your trade will be a good supply of books on the advantages of a vegetarian diet, a good supply of recipes and cookbooks, and an invitation to share a meal. Consider lending a book to your family doctor, teacher, or minister and then asking them how they liked it a few weeks later. In doing so, you will be planting seeds that may take time to take root, so be patient.

It takes time for change to happen. Always remember how long it took to change the world's attitude toward smoking cigarettes. It took fifty years from the surgeon general announcing that cigarette smoking is bad for your health until society really got the message the way it does today. Your parents' generation has given you a head start. Now it's up to you to bring it across the finish line.

CHAPTER 8

What Should I Eat?

What should vegetarians eat?

Here's the secret formula: Vegetarians should base their diet around five key food groups: fruits, vegetables, whole grains, legumes (beans), and nuts and seeds. As long as you eat a variety of different foods from each of these groups, you should get all the nutrition you need. The diagram below shows the relative importance of each group. Aim to get several portions of vegetables and at least three portions each of whole grains, fruits, and legumes every day. Nuts and seeds are healthy foods, but it's easy to eat too much of these—three good-sized handfuls a week are sufficient.

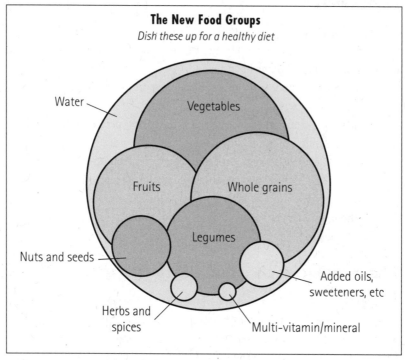

Figure 12. A healthy vegetarian eats a variety of foods.

Don't forget your nutritional insurance. Life often gets busy and we can't always pay as much attention to our diet as we need to, so we also recommend that you take a good multivitamin-mineral supplement. Make sure that it contains vitamin B_{12} and vitamin D.

Be smart with spices. Use herbs and spices to add flavor and variety to your food, but go easy on the salt since it can raise your blood pressure and force your kidneys to work overtime.

It's fine to eat moderate amounts of vegetable oils and natural sweeteners when called for in recipes. Evaporated cane juice, maple syrup, rice syrup, and agave nectar are better choices than refined sugar or artificial sweeteners. Don't forget that chocolate is a vegetarian product, and dark chocolate, in small amounts, is particularly healthful because of its antioxidant properties.

Scientists aren't kidding when they say that our bodies are mostly made up of water. Water is an important component of a balanced diet. Aim for at least six to eight cups a day.

What are some examples of foods in the key food groups?

Here's a list of some familiar foods in each key food group:

Fruits: apples, bananas, blueberries, cantaloupes, grapes, peaches, pears, raspberries, strawberries, and watermelon

Legumes (beans): black beans, chickpeas, green beans, lentils, peanuts, peas, soybeans, and soy products (including tofu)

Nuts and seeds: almonds, cashews, flax seeds, pecans, pumpkin seeds, sesame seeds, sunflower seeds, and walnuts

Vegetables: bell peppers, broccoli, cabbage, carrots, cauliflower, cucumbers, eggplant, kale, lettuce, okra, potatoes, pumpkins, sweet potatoes, tomatoes, yams, and zucchini

Whole grains: barley, brown rice, corn, oatmeal, quinoa, whole-grain bread, and whole-grain pasta

What familiar meals include these food groups?

You might think, "Help; I don't eat any of these key foods right now!" but you'd be surprised how easy it can be. Think of a bean burrito. It includes beans, vegetables (as salad), and often whole grains in the wrap. So in a simple burrito you get three of the food groups covered. A veggie burger on a whole-grain bun with some salad will similarly cover three of the key food groups. A baked sweet potato with baked beans and sweet corn is an easy meal to make at home. It also includes three of the food groups. Soy products (made from soybeans) are the basis of many veggie burgers and other meat substitute products, so look for these in your grocery store as a great way to get a serving or two of legumes into your diet.

Simple snacks can easily help you meet your need for the other groups: fresh fruit, fruit smoothies, granola, and trail mix are all easy to eat when you're on the go.

Why are there no dairy or eggs in the key food groups?

You'll notice that there is no dairy or egg food group in the diagram on page 77. That's because we don't consider dairy products or eggs to be necessary in your vegetarian diet (see pages 14, 15, and 44 for more information on this). Do your best to keep these foods to a minimum, ideally cutting them out altogether. There are many good alternatives to cow's milk, which you can use on cereal, to drink, or for cooking. Give soymilk, almond milk, or rice milk a try, and look for soy or coconut ice cream and yogurt. Try a tofu scramble instead of eggs, and some soy, rice, or almond cheese instead of cheese made from cow's milk.

What are whole foods and why are they important?

Go for whole foods whenever possible. These are foods that are eaten as close to their natural state (how they grew) as possible. It's much less likely that damaging trans fats, sugars and artificial sweeteners, artificial colors and flavors, or other chemicals will have been added to your food if it is in a natural state. For instance, whole pinto beans are usually better than refried beans, tofu is better than a processed veggie burger, and home-baked cookies are better than most store-bought ones. But no one is perfect. We all have busy lives and we often have to make compromises. Beans in any form are a more healthful source of protein in a burrito than pieces of beef or chicken. A veggie burger is much better for you than a hamburger. If you can't find unprocessed choices easily, meat-free ones of any kind are still much better for you than meat-based choices.

What's wrong with junk food as long as it's vegetarian?

You deserve better than junk food. Some young people choose to go vegetarian without regard for their health. They might base their diet on french fries, Twinkies, and Coca Cola, which is technically speaking a vegetarian diet, but this is not recommended. A diet based on junk food, while it could be vegetarian, is low in important nutrients and not good for your body. Sooner or later you will get sick from this kind of diet. If you want to convince people that you're making a responsible choice, then make sure to include as little junk food in your diet as you possibly can—preferably none. Junk food includes deep-fried foods such as french fries, onion rings, most potato chips; sugary foods such as candy, cakes, cookies, and cereals (unless they're made from whole grains and include very little sugar); white bread; and soda pop.

So remember the five key food groups. Choose almost all of the food you eat or drink from these groups, and ensure that it's as natural and unprocessed as possible. Take a multivitamin-mineral supplement every day and wash it all down with plenty of water. That's what a healthy vegetarian eats.

Where do vegetarians get their protein from?

The simple answer is that vegetarians get all the protein they need from plant foods. Most Americans have been trained to believe that the only sources of protein are meat, poultry, fish, dairy, and eggs. It's true that all these foods have a lot of protein, but you may be surprised to learn that many vegetables, whole grains, legumes (beans), nuts, and seeds have lots of protein, too. The Food and Nutrition Board of the National Research Council states that you need to get 8 to 10 percent of your calories from protein. Take a look at this chart of vegetables, legumes, nuts, and seeds, and you'll see that if you include plenty of these kinds of foods in your diet, you can't get less than 8 to 10 percent of your calories as protein:

Table 3. Protein in plant foods

Vegetables	Protein*	Legumes and grains	Protein*
spinach	49%	lentils	29%
broccoli	45%	pinto beans	26%
kale	45%	chickpeas	23%
mushroom	39%	peanuts	18%
okra	27%	sunflower seeds	17%
tomato	20%	wheat berries	17%
pumpkin	15%	oatmeal, cooked	15%
corn	15%	cashews	12%
potato	11%	brown rice	8%

Source: Keith Akers, *A Vegetarian Sourcebook* (Denver: Vegetarian Press, 1993).
*Protein is shown as a percentage of calories.

If you remove the outer skin or shell from a grain or a vegetable, you may lose some of the protein, as well as some of the fiber and vitamins. This is one reason why whole wheat flour is better than white flour, brown rice is better than white rice, and a baked potato in its skin is better than mashed potatoes, for example.

The key point to remember is that you can easily get all the protein you need from plant foods, and in fact the biggest problem most people have with protein is getting too much of it, rather than too little.

Is it necessary to combine plant foods in a meal to get "complete protein"?

Don't fall for protein myths. The idea that you have to combine plant proteins is a myth that was popularized back in the 1960s and '70s. Dietitians now know that our bodies can store the amino acids that make up protein for a few days, so as long as you eat a range of different foods over the course of a day or two, you will get all the protein you need.

Let's talk science for a bit. Amino acids are the building blocks that are strung together in different combinations to make up the different proteins that we eat. Eight of these amino acids are essential to have in our diet, since our bodies can't synthesize them. All foods that contain protein include some of each of these amino acids, but the amount of each amino acid varies from one type of food to the next. So if you only ate potatoes, but ate a huge amount of them, you would eventually get all the amino acids you need. Obviously it's easier, and much healthier, to eat a range of foods in order to get the full set of essential amino acids without eating excessive quantities. The key point here is that an amino acid is exactly the same regardless of whether it comes from a plant or an animal.

Now let's do some comparison shopping. If you buy animal proteins you're going to face a high price tag, and we're not just talking money. While animal products do contain all eight essential amino acids, they come with a high price tag of cholesterol, saturated fats, and carcinogens (cancer-causing chemicals). Plant proteins come with no cholesterol, are low in saturated fat, and are high in fiber and other cancer-fighting nutrients. That makes plant proteins a much better deal.

Remember that most meat eaters actually are getting too much protein. A diet too high in protein strains the kidneys, and animal protein has also been linked to osteoporosis (weak and brittle bones). So the best way to get all the different amino acids you need is to eat a wide range of vegetables, whole grains, and especially beans and nuts.

What about soyfoods?

Many people may have heard rumors about soy causing all kinds of health and hormonal problems. Don't believe them! Soy products are perfectly nutritious and have been eaten for thousands of years by billions of people. These rumors, such as that it will cause homosexuality or breast cancer, have no basis in science whatsoever, and most were started by a single organization, which just happens to be funded by the meat industry. In fact, numerous scientific studies have shown that soy won't make men gay or impotent and that women who eat the most soy have the lowest rates of breast cancer. Soy has been shown to lower the rates of heart disease, type 2 diabetes, and osteoporosis. Science says soy is safe!

Can I eat chicken and still be a vegetarian?

A vegetarian, by definition, does not eat meat, fish, or fowl, so if you eat chicken you are not a vegetarian. Many people who want to be vegetarians start by cutting out red meat. That's a great first step. Any reduction in the amount of meat you eat is better for your health, for the animals, and for the environment. But chicken has about as much cholesterol and saturated fat as beef, and eating it gives rise to many of the same health and environmental problems as eating red meat. Chickens also often live miserable lives before being killed for their meat, so compassion for animals gives vegetarians another good reason not to eat chicken.

Can I eat fish if I'm a vegetarian?

Some fish eaters like to call themselves vegetarian, but a fish eater is not a vegetarian any more than is someone who eats chicken. It is definitely a step in the right direction to cut out beef, pork, and chicken, even if you still eat fish. But fish are no better for our health than meat, and the fishing industry causes huge amounts of damage to the oceans and the fish that live in them.

What many people don't realize is that fish contains about as much cholesterol as meat. It also contains some saturated fat. Since dietary cholesterol, along with saturated fat, is a major cause of heart disease, and the most common cause of death in America is a heart attack, fish is not a good addition to our diets. Not only that, but many fish contain toxic chemicals, such as mercury, PCBs, and dioxins. These chemicals are produced by industry and wind up in our streams and rivers. They are washed out to sea and absorbed into the organisms that fish feed upon. These chemicals are then absorbed into the fishes' bodies and stay there for a long time. Bigger fish eat the smaller ones and so accumulate even more of these chemicals. Tuna, being one of the bigger fish at the top of the food chain, has much more of these chemicals than smaller fish, and it is now recommended that young children and pregnant women don't eat tuna more than once a week because of the risk of mercury poisoning. Many of these toxic chemicals are thought to have links to cancer, so we recommend eating no fish at all.

There has been much talk about fish having omega-3 fatty acids in their fat, and that you can't get your essential fatty acids anywhere else. Don't fall for this fish tale. In fact, the best sources of omega-3 fatty acids are flaxseeds and oil, walnuts, soy products, and canola oil. If you use canola oil regularly for cooking, and eat walnuts and flaxseeds from time to time, you will get all the omega-3 fatty acids you need.

Don't I need to eat dairy products?

Wipe the milk off your mustache! The dairy industry would have you believe that milk is an essential part of your diet and that your bones won't get enough calcium without it. This message has been pushed so much, and over such a long period of time, that most Americans take it as a given, and for many years the government included dairy as an essential food group. But in fact, plant foods provide all the calcium you need, and getting it from plant foods has several advantages.

Take a moment and rethink consuming dairy products. Do you know of any animals other than humans that drink milk after they've been weaned off their mother's milk? Come to that, do you know of any other animal that drinks the milk of another species of animal? It just doesn't happen in nature. Gorillas and elephants alike are able to build strong healthy bones on plants alone, and so can we.

Milk is a global nonstarter. Dairy consumption is rare in many other parts of the world. East Asians and Africans generally don't consume any dairy products, and they have fewer cases of osteoporosis (weak and brittle bones) than people in the West. In fact most people of East Asian or African descent are lactose intolerant, which means that their bodies don't digest milk products well, and they often get symptoms such as gas, diarrhea, or stomach cramps from consuming milk. People of European origin are less likely to be lactose intolerant, but that doesn't necessarily mean that milk is good for them. Finland has the highest per capita consumption of dairy products in the world. It is also the country with one of the highest levels of several serious diseases, including heart disease and diabetes. Finnish officials are looking into the reasons for this, and are starting to notice that there's a strong connection between the amount of dairy products consumed and levels of type 1 diabetes in particular.

Milk became popular as a source of food because it is high in protein and fat. In cold climates in the winter, poor peasants found it to be an invaluable source of nutrition when there was little else available. Today, with modern refrigeration and transportation, it is rare for people in the developed world to suffer from a lack of basic nutrients. As we've already stated, most Americans suffer from eating too much protein, not too little. One look at the wide selection of low-fat dairy products on store shelves shows that we know how bad the saturated fat in milk is for our health. But we need to recognize that the cholesterol in milk isn't good for us either, and that milk contains higher levels of industrial and agricultural toxins, which increase the risk of cancer.

We've got a bone to pick with the dairy industry, which tries to emphasize the calcium in milk now that they've taken it on the chin for saturated fat and cholesterol. Scientific studies show that milk doesn't prevent osteoporosis. While cow's milk does contain calcium, in fact it doesn't help keep our bones strong, both because it is not well absorbed, and because it is high in acidic amino acids, which counteract the calcium.

While we're on the subject, cola-style drinks can also counteract calcium in the diet and in the bones. These drinks contain high levels of phosphoric acid, which needs to be neutralized by using calcium from our bones. So don't think that you can drink soda instead of milk. Neither will help build strong bones, and soda drinks actually cause harm. Drink water to avoid these problems, or try calcium-fortified orange juice or milk alternatives such as soymilk and rice milk for some extra calcium.

Which plant foods contain calcium?

Take a look at this chart, which shows how much calcium different plant foods contain, and how much of the calcium is absorbed when we consume that food. You'll see that there are many sources of calcium other than dairy products, and that the absorption rate is much higher than dairy for many of those foods.

Table 4. Calcium content of various foods

Food	Calcium, in milligrams*	Percentage of calcium absorbed
bok choy	870	53
collard greens	609	not available
orange juice (calcium fortified)	320	52
tofu, set with calcium	287	31
kale	270	49
green leaf lettuce	240	not available
broccoli	215	61
cow's milk (for comparison)	188	32
sesame seeds	170	21
cabbage	160	65
white beans	72	22
molasses	71	not available

Source: USDA National Nutrient Database.   *Calcium amount per 100-calorie serving.

Be sure to include green vegetables, such as collards, kale, broccoli, and cabbage in your diet if you can. These vegetables are packed with calcium, iron, fiber, and many other valuable nutrients.

Should I eat eggs?

Eggs are not all they're cracked up to be, and are not necessary in a vegetarian diet. There are many good reasons to avoid them. Eggs have more cholesterol than any other food, so avoiding eggs is a great way to reduce your cholesterol levels. They also contain some saturated fat. Eggs are also renowned as breeding grounds for salmonella, and tend to accumulate the antibiotics that have been fed to the chickens to keep them free of diseases. These antibiotics are not good for our bodies.

There are many great substitutes for eggs, which can be used in your favorite recipes. Try a tofu scramble in place of eggs for breakfast. Use baking soda to make your cake rise, and tofu, mashed bananas, or ground flaxseeds to replace the moisture from eggs in a baking recipe.

How will I get enough iron in my diet?

A wide variety of plant foods contain all the iron you need. Iron is an essential component of our red blood cells, used to carry oxygen around the body. While adult men typically don't need very much iron, growing children, menstruating and especially pregnant women do need more. People often think that vegetarians don't get enough iron since meat contains iron, but studies show that vegetarians have no more likelihood of anemia (iron deficiency) than nonvegetarians. Beans and lentils, tomatoes, watermelon, and green leafy vegetables such as kale are particularly good sources of iron, better than meat on a per-calorie basis, and don't come packaged with cholesterol and high amounts of saturated fat.

What is fiber and why is it important?

Fiber is the indigestible part of plant foods, and most people just don't get enough of it. You might think that if it's indigestible, fiber is of no use to us, but in fact it's essential in helping us to form stools and pass them out of our bodies quickly and efficiently. When we don't eat enough fiber we can become constipated, and chronic constipation can lead to more serious conditions, such as hemorrhoids, appendicitis, and diverticulosis. By age sixty, two-thirds of Americans have diverticulosis, a disease where little pockets form in the colon; these pockets can become infected, making a trip to the hospital necessary.

There's no fiber in meat. All animal products, such as meat, fish, dairy, and eggs contain no fiber at all. The same is true for most highly processed foods, such as white bread, cookies, cakes, and candy. But all fruits, vegetables, whole grains, and legumes contain plenty of fiber, so vegetarians who eat a wholesome diet don't suffer from any of these problems. By moving your bowels at least once a day, you'll stay healthier and be able to avoid these problems. Eating lots of whole grains, fruits, and vegetables, and drinking plenty of water, will help ensure that this happens.

If I wanted to just choose a few plant foods to get started, which are the best nutritionally?

It is best to include a variety of fruits, vegetables, grains, nuts, and legumes in your diet, but some give you more antioxidants, vitamins, and minerals per serving than others. Here's a selection of the best foods to eat:

Fruits: blueberries, pears, watermelon
Grains: corn, quinoa, wheat germ, and whole wheat
Legumes: black beans, peas, red lentils, and tofu
Nuts and seeds: almonds, flaxseeds, and walnuts
Vegetables: broccoli, kale, okra, sweet potatoes, and tomatoes

What are organic foods and are they important?

Who needs all the pesticides routinely sprayed on conventional crops? Organic plant foods are grown without artificial pesticides and fertilizers. Farmers must meet strict standards in order for their crops to be certified organic. For processed foods, more than 95 percent of the ingredients have to be organic for the product to be able to be called organic, and there must be no artificial ingredients. For animal foods, the animal has to have been fed exclusively on organic feed and not given antibiotics or growth hormones throughout its life.

Good planets are hard to find, so let's take care of the one we have! Producing organic foods is much less damaging to the environment, so choosing organic food of any kind is a good thing to do, since it encourages farmers to grow more organic foods. Because organic crops do not contain pesticides or herbicides, they are safer for the farm workers who raise and harvest them, as well as safer for you to eat. Organic animal products are also safer, to some degree, because the animals have been fed organic crops.

One thing to bear in mind: while choosing organic products will help you avoid pesticides or herbicides, there are industrial chemicals, such as mercury, dioxin, and PCBs, that are found in organic products as well as conventional food. These are carried in the air and water and can settle on any foods, including organic ones. They are also often dumped into streams that are used for irrigating crops and feeding animals, whether they are organic or not.

Most of our pesticide and toxic chemical exposure comes from animal foods, not plant foods. This is because animals store and concentrate these toxic chemicals in their bodies over their lifetime. When you eat the animal you get the toxins it's been storing up just for you. By going vegetarian, or even better yet vegan, you'll cut out most of your exposure to these dangerous chemicals.

Choosing organic foods takes you a little further along the path to safer food. Organic foods do tend to be more expensive than conventional foods, but if you can afford it, choosing organic foods wherever possible will limit your exposure to some toxic chemicals and help the environment. Avoiding animal products, whether organic or not, will reduce your exposure to all toxic chemicals, and will cost you less.

There are some foods I can't eat. Can I still be a vegetarian?

Don't worry, vegetarian diets can be very adaptable. If you suffer from allergies or sensitivities to certain foods, you may think that you have enough to deal with, without having to try to give up meat or other animal products as well. However, it is usually possible to find plenty of foods to enjoy a balanced vegetarian diet. No one food is essential to a nutritious vegetarian diet—the variety of plant foods available means that you can forgo several of them without any trouble at all.

Some allergies or intolerances are very common. For example 95 percent of people of African or East Asian descent have trouble digesting dairy products, and they often find that their health improves dramatically when they give up eating these foods. There are many alternative milks to try, such as soy, almond, rice, or oat milk. Nondairy ice cream and yogurt are very tasty and enable you to enjoy the tastes you love without consuming dairy. Nondairy cheeses often still include casein, a milk protein, to help them melt. Lactose-intolerant people are able to tolerate casein, because the lactose has been removed, but those with dairy allergies will need to look for the cheeselike products that don't include casein. The solution is to read the labels carefully.

Other sensitivities to products such as soy, nuts, or wheat are not common, but avoiding these products can make a big difference to the well-being of the individual concerned. To avoid soy in a vegetarian diet, focus on eating other legumes, as well as a wide variety of fruits, vegetables, and whole grains. Lentils are particularly easy to digest, and not likely to cause anyone problems. You may find that you can tolerate some forms of soyfoods; tempeh for example, is easily digested because it is a fermented product.

People trying to avoid wheat or gluten products can experiment with other grains. Quinoa is a particularly useful food, as it is easy to cook and contains no gluten. Pasta made from quinoa is available in natural food stores. Rice and corn are other grains that work for some people with wheat or gluten intolerance.

Nuts and peanuts (which are legumes) are great sources of protein and healthful fats, making them excellent additions to a vegetarian diet. Some people are allergic to these foods, however, and are unable to risk eating even a small amount of them. If you can't eat nuts or peanuts, beans and seeds (if you are not allergic to them), such as flaxseeds, sesame seeds, and sunflower seeds, are tasty options that provide similar nutritional value.

Some people, and especially some alternative health-care providers, jump to the conclusion that a food allergy or intolerance is the cause of a health issue, based on little real evidence. When it comes to nutrition, science provides the best guidance. Make sure your allergy or intolerance is based on reliable medical tests before making any significant decisions.

What else should I make sure to include in my diet?

A nutritious vegetarian diet based on fruits, vegetables, grains, legumes, nuts, and seeds, in theory should provide all the nutrition you need. Indeed, many people have lived all their lives, and even through several generations, on a vegetarian diet, without paying too much attention to particular nutrients, and have remained very healthy. But today people live busy lives, and don't have the time or the opportunity to get the variety of nutrition they need every day. A multivitamin-mineral supplement can help ensure you're getting all you need.

Be sure that your vitamins include both vitamin B_{12} and vitamin D. Vegans need to make sure that they have a source of vitamin B_{12} in their diet, because modern food processing methods remove even small amounts of soil from the food we eat, and vitamin B_{12}, which is found in the soil, is also removed. Animals store up some vitamin B_{12}, which they pass on to us if we eat their products. But if you're following a vegetarian diet that is also free of eggs and dairy products, you need to get some supplementation for vitamin B_{12}.

The sun doesn't always shine. Vitamin D is made by the action of sunlight on the skin. However, many people who live in northern latitudes don't get much sun exposure, and others use sunblock all the time to prevent overexposure, so they may not be getting as much vitamin D as they need, whether they are vegetarian or not. Some foods are fortified with vitamin D, but it has been found to be the most common vitamin deficiency among the American population, so we recommend that everyone take additional vitamin D.

A good multivitamin-mineral supplement will give you the vitamins B_{12} and D you may need, and will cover all the other vitamins and minerals as well. This is a good idea for everyone, whether vegetarian or not. There's no need to shell out big money for these. The generic will do just fine and megadoses are unnecessary.

CHAPTER 9

Dealing with Family, Friends, and Others

How can I get my parents to agree to my becoming a vegetarian?

If you're living with your parents and you are dependent on them for your living expenses and food, you need to be very diplomatic when approaching them about your desire to go vegetarian. You know your parents, but you may not be able to predict how they will react to this subject if it hasn't come up in discussions before. The key is to stay calm, and be prepared for the questions that may arise by educating yourself as thoroughly as possible.

The trick is to try to understand things from your parent's point of view. Some parents may think that young people make irresponsible and impulsive decisions. Here are some simple steps you should be prepared to take:

> If you've made irresponsible decisions in the past, own up to them and explain why this decision is different.

> Emphasize that this isn't just a passing phase, and that you're not being impulsive.

> Show that you've thought it through carefully, that you really want to do it, and that it's something you plan to do for the long term.

> Explain that you understand the importance of eating healthfully, that you won't be just eating french fries and drinking Coke, but that you have a plan to eat plenty of nutritious foods, such as fruits and vegetables.

> State that you feel this is a very responsible decision, and that you're asking for their help in carrying it through.

The questions below have come up for many other young people. If you stay calm and give clear, well-informed answers, chances are, your parents will listen. They will respect your decision and do what they can to help.

How can I show my parents that this is a wise choice?

Facts have force, but when it comes to parenting, fear for the safety of their children can be just as powerful. Food is a very emotive issue for many people, and your parents are likely to be no different. They may feel afraid that this is a fad diet and that you are going to become unhealthy. If you have read this book thoroughly, and you have it at hand when talking with your parents, you'll be able to show them some of the facts. Ask them to be specific in what they worry about, such as that you won't get enough protein, then show them the relevant answer in the book and let them read it for themselves. Show them the statement from the American Dietetic Association on page 22, as this may help to reassure them. They may need time to think and read more about it, so don't rush them to give you an answer right away.

My parents think it's too complicated. How can I reassure them that I can do it?

Many parents are busy people and they like meals to be simple and straightforward. Having one person in the family eat differently from the others makes it more complicated. They may not have the time or inclination to learn new recipes, look for new foods, and to try to make meals that incorporate your wishes.

Be the change you want to see. Since you are the one who wants to make a change, you have to be willing to help. Look through vegetarian cookbooks, websites, and magazines for ideas on what you could eat and how it would fit with other family members' requirements. Go grocery shopping, read the ingredient labels, look at the prices, and help choose the foods you'd like to eat. You may need to try some new foods and start some new habits, such as helping with the cooking. Being helpful and open-minded will make a big difference in helping your parents become comfortable with the idea of you being vegetarian.

How can I reassure my parents that it won't be too expensive?

Do the math and cost it out for them. When you are a vegetarian, you have many choices as to how you eat, just as when you're a meat eater. There is no reason for food to be any more expensive for a vegetarian than for a meat eater, and you may well be able to save money. It's possible to eat out expensively or cheaply, and similarly when eating at home you can cook simple ingredients from scratch, or buy somewhat more expensive prepared meals.

Jump on the learning curve and get a good cookbook. If you learn to cook basic ingredients, such as pasta, grains, and beans, use herbs and spices for flavoring, and include plenty of fresh vegetables, you will be eating inexpensively and in the healthiest way possible. You may be able to buy basic ingredients from bulk bins in a natural food store, and buy fresh vegetables at a farmers' market to keep the costs down even further. If you buy prepared foods that you put straight into the microwave, the costs will be a little higher than self-prepared meals. So the best way to keep the costs to a minimum is to buy a suitable cookbook and learn to cook nutritious meals for yourself.

Check out the grocery store. If someone else usually does the cooking for you, and you want that to continue, we suggest that you visit the grocery store together and look at the prices of foods that can be incorporated into the family meals or easily prepared by you separately.

For only a few dollars more you can buy quality. Your parents may be willing to pay a little more if they see the value of it. If your diet has been focused on extremely cheap "junk food" in the past, then starting to eat fresh fruits and vegetables may cause your overall food bill to increase. You can tell them to think of this as an investment in your health, and the benefit will be seen in a reduction in your medical bills in the long term.

How can I show them that this idea isn't just brainwashing?

"Help! My kids have been kidnapped by vegetarians and brainwashed!" This could be how some parents react. They may have developed an image of vegetarians from the media, which sometimes imply that all vegetarians are weird. Others may have come across an extreme vegetarian group in the past, which gave them a poor impression of all vegetarians. If you suspect that this is a cause of their fears, you may want to mention that the common stereotypes about vegetarians are not very realistic, and that many ordinary people are vegetarian; they just don't get into the news. You can also talk about the people in history who were vegetarian, such as Albert Einstein and Ben Franklin, whom your parents are likely to respect.

"Mom, meet my vegetarian friends!" If you first learned about going meatless because one of your friends is vegetarian, it may be a good idea for your parents to meet the friend before you raise the issue of becoming vegetarian. They are more likely to trust someone they have gotten to know. You can also show them reliable sources of information, such as this book, to help them see that it's not just your friend's wacky idea.

What if my parents think I don't love them anymore?

No one wants his or her love rejected. For many parents, feeding you was the way that they first expressed their love for you. Some parents may take it personally, thinking that you don't love them, if you won't eat their cooking. If you get a sense that this is an issue, you need to reassure them that you still love them, and that you appreciate every effort they make to provide you with meals that you enjoy. It's just that since you've learned more about the harm caused by eating animal products, the foods you enjoy have changed.

What if my parents worry about my being teased?

Words can hurt. If your parents are concerned that you'll be teased, or that it will be difficult for you in some other way, you can reassure them that you'd rather be yourself and be true to what you believe in, and get teased, than be someone you're not just to fit in. You can acknowledge that you may have limited food choices at times, but that you're willing to cook your own food, or bring your own food to a social event, so that you always have good food you feel comfortable eating.

What can I do if my parents won't let me be vegetarian?

If you don't succeed in convincing your parents at your first attempt, don't be discouraged. Staying calm is vital, especially if your parents' reaction is anything but calm. The temptation may be to yell or scream back at them, but a better way to go is to say, "I can see that it's going to take you a while to get comfortable with the idea, so maybe we could discuss this again another day."

Be patient. It is likely that you'll need to take time to show them that you are really serious about your decision, that it's not just a phase you're going through, that you have researched the facts and that you are willing to make a consistent effort to eat healthfully. If you continue to eat your parents' cooking, leaving out the nonvegetarian parts, and then grumble about the food choices available to you at home, your diet will not be particularly healthful, and you won't earn their respect. However, if you offer to cook meals for the family a few times a week, they may well compromise and cook adaptable meals that work well for you and the rest of the family.

Rome wasn't built in a day. If you are able to buy your own food and cook separately, over time your parents will probably get used to the idea of you eating vegetarian food, and start to become curious about what you're eating. With patience and diligence, you'll find they'll become more flexible and you'll be able to enjoy family meals together again.

You might not want to hear this, but in some situations you may have to wait until you are older to switch to a vegetarian diet. If your parents are insistent upon you continuing to eat meat, and you are not old enough or financially independent enough to buy your own food, you may just have to live with the situation until you are free to make your own food choices. But continuing to draw your parents' attention to any articles or books on the health benefits of vegetarian diets from time to time may bring them around eventually.

How will my friends react?

Know your facts well and you'll do better with your friends. Many young people are curious about different ways of living. They will no doubt have many questions, some of which may seem silly to you; but if you know your facts and are patient about repeating the same answers to many different people, they will respect you for it. Friends can be very accepting, as long as you are clear about why you've decided to change what you eat.

Others can be a pain, but there are ways to deal with them too. Some people, usually not your friends, may hear about you being vegetarian and use the information to tease or make jokes. It is best to be good-natured about the teasing, to laugh along with them, and then correct any factual errors in what they said by saying "Actually, from what I've read it appears that..." Arguing or getting angry about what they've said is rarely effective and can make you look insecure.

We've heard it all before. One common comment you may get goes something like this: "Look how I'm eating this delicious steak, yum, yum. Doesn't it make you jealous?" Your answer could be something like, "I can eat meat if I want, but I choose not to," "I've really lost my taste for meat since going vegetarian," "I'm glad it's your arteries you're clogging, not mine," or "I don't tell you what to eat, so please let me eat what I choose." But it's often best just to ignore critical comments and jokes—they'll probably stop sooner if they don't get a good response.

Don't lose your cool. The important thing is to remain relaxed and respectful at all times. Other people are entitled to eat whatever they like, and so are you. So don't get on your soapbox and start criticizing their food, preaching about factory farms, animal cruelty, global warming, or anything else—that's the fastest way to make people feel overwhelmed and defensive.

Actions speak even louder than words. Live by example. Unfortunately, "radical and pushy" is a stereotype that people sometimes connect with vegetarians, so it is even more important not to fall into that trap. Just answer questions simply when asked. Then your friends and acquaintances will see that you haven't changed, that you're a normal person who just happens to choose to be vegetarian.

How can I answer why I went vegetarian without offending someone?

Stay positive and respectful. When someone asks you about being a vegetarian, it's important to show that it's a positive decision and that you enjoy eating this way, especially if you hope to influence other people to become vegetarian themselves someday. Here are some suggestions for what to say:

> ➤ "You'd be amazed at how many health benefits there are from eating this way."
> ➤ "When I learned about how the animals are treated on most factory farms, I couldn't bring myself to eat meat any more."
> ➤ "You probably haven't heard too much about this, but in fact the raising of animals is very damaging to the environment, so I wanted to do something to help."

Don't get negative. If you give a negative or boring impression of eating vegetarian food, you can be sure that they will be put off for a very long time. Many people are also turned off by scary or horrific images, so it is usually counterproductive to say anything along the lines of the following:

> ➤ "Let me tell you all about the horrible diseases you're going to get by eating meat."
> ➤ "Here's some gruesome pictures of how animals are treated on factory farms."
> ➤ "People who eat meat are responsible for global warming, water pollution, burning down the rainforest, and even global hunger. How could you live with that on your conscience?"

Don't come on too strong. Some people just can't handle food issues. The most important thing to avoid is overwhelming a person. If they stop asking questions, or don't show an interest in the subject, then move right along to a totally different topic. Sometimes the message takes a few months or even a few years to sink in, after planting the seed.

What do I say to those who say "I would be vegetarian too, but . . ."?

You might see it in your friends' faces—a guilty conscience. Many people may feel guilty about eating meat. They start making excuses and the excuses are endless. Just remind them that you used to feel that way, too, and explain how you worked through it. For example, many people make the excuse that they couldn't give up chicken, so you can explain that there are so many good meat alternatives these days, they'd never know the difference. You can tell them what it was that inspired you to change your diet—maybe a book, an article, a friend, or just a realization. Hearing why someone changed their diet can be very inspiring.

What do you recommend when going out with friends or to parties?

Do some advance research and come prepared. When you're going out to eat with friends, encourage them to pick a restaurant that you know has some veggie options you can choose. It might help to look up the restaurant online to see what menu items are OK for you to eat. Even if you aren't able to influence the choice of restaurant, you may be able to ask the kitchen to make something special if you can't find a suitable meal on the menu. Most chefs and restaurants don't mind special orders, so it's important to speak up. Another alternative is to eat beforehand, and just go along to enjoy the company.

Know before you go. At a catered dinner, ask (beforehand if possible) whether the caterer has any vegetarian options. When going to a private party, it's a good idea to mention to the host that you are vegetarian, so that they can cater for your needs if food is to be provided. Alternatively, you can just ask which dishes include meat when you arrive, so that you can be sure to avoid them, rather than putting your host to any special trouble.

Some people just need a little help. You might want to offer to bring some food, so that you know you'll have something to eat. At a barbecue, bring a package of veggie burgers or veggie hot dogs for the grill. A potluck is a great opportunity to show others how delicious vegetarian food can be, so it's worth making a special effort to bring a particularly appetizing dish or two. You can pick something up from the deli counter at a natural food store if you don't wish to cook. Be sure to eat when you first arrive, since others may like your food so much that they eat it all before you get any!

How can I turn down Grandma's turkey dinner?

Grandma is not really serving turkey. She's serving love and it's way more important to make her feel loved in return than to eat her turkey. Even so, holidays can be a challenge, since the big family meal is often the focus of the whole holiday. The most important thing to your family is that you are present, warm, and friendly. If your vegetarianism is still a new idea, you may need to let people know very gently. You could say, "Don't go to any special trouble. I'll just eat the side dishes." At a big dinner, you'll probably find plenty to eat, but if you know that the stuffing will be cooked inside the turkey and the beans will be cooked with bacon, then you may wish to bring something else to eat. If it would break Grandma's heart for you not to eat her turkey, then you may just have to take a very small portion, and remember that this only happens once a year. Plenty of people think of themselves as vegetarian while making the occasional compromise to avoid hurting those they love the most.

Can I kiss a meat eater?

There are no hard and fast rules for who vegetarians can kiss. If you love every aspect of a person except what they choose to eat, then you may well decide that they should eat their food and you eat yours, and both of you can just accept the situation. We know many couples who have lived together happily for many years with this arrangement. Over time, the meat-eating partner may become comfortable with eating vegetarian all the time or at least most of the time, just choosing a meat dish in a restaurant once in a while—or he or she may continue to insist on meat at every meal. Either way is OK if you're OK with it.

But what if you're not OK with it? Some people feel that their food choices are so important to them that they can't face the idea of dating someone who eats meat. You are entitled to make that choice, but be aware that at present the percentage of vegetarians in the general population is very small, so it may take a little more work to find a boyfriend or girlfriend. You can try attending vegetarian dinners and get-togethers, or looking online for veggie dates.

Just remember that there are many open-minded people out there who just haven't heard about the benefits of a vegetarian diet. They could be happy to learn about becoming vegetarian in a warm and supportive environment. It's better not to deprive them of kisses until they become vegetarian, or they'll be out the door in no time, and you'll be back to square one.

How should I tell my date that I'm vegetarian?

Be up front about it. They'll find out soon enough anyway. When you first start dating someone (let's assume it's a "him" for ease of writing, but these suggestions work for women too), you may be nervous as to how he will react to the idea that you're a vegetarian. The key is to be honest about it, but not make it too big of a deal.

Avoid problems. You probably don't want him to invite you out to a steakhouse for dinner, so make sure that he knows you're vegetarian before your first meal out together. If your first date is at a restaurant, you might have to mention your dietary preferences right away, but ideally wait until you can bring up the subject in casual conversation.

Gently raise the issue. You might start by asking what kinds of foods he likes to eat. This will give you an idea of how flexible and open-minded he might be to your eating choices. Whatever you do, don't belittle his food choices: you want him to respect your choices, so you must respect his. It's a two-way street.

Now it's your turn to mention that you happen to be a vegetarian. Hopefully he'll be equally respectful about your choices. If he isn't, then you may have to gently point this out to him. He could have lots of questions at this point. Remember that many people just don't know anything about this way of eating, so keep your answers short and respectful.

It's decision time. Based on his reaction, you can decide whether you want to continue the relationship, but remember that he may just need time to get used to the idea. For now, you know that he knows, and you can focus on discovering the many other interests you do have in common.

How will my doctor react?

Medical researchers rave about vegetarian diets, but many family doctors have meat stuck in their ears and don't seem to be able to hear the message. While this is now definitely starting to change, it may take a few more years for some doctors to get used to the idea that a vegetarian diet is the healthiest way to go.

To make matters worse, most doctors have had very little, if any, training in nutrition. Others are aware of the benefits of following a vegetarian diet but don't want to risk losing patients by routinely suggesting it. The thing to remember is that meat eating is currently at the stage that cigarette smoking was fifty years ago. It is more socially acceptable to eat meat than not to, most doctors still eat meat themselves, and so they may not be comfortable with telling their patients not to eat meat.

Don't walk in to your doctor's office empty-handed. Bring the statement by the American Dietetic Association (see page 22). This may help your doctor to become comfortable with the idea. If you are healthy, he or she will probably accept your food choices, but they may not be particularly supportive. Don't be surprised if your doctor orders some blood tests when he hears that you're vegetarian. He may be practicing defensive medicine fearing the occasional lawsuit, or he may just be ignorant. This is a good time to mention that you take a daily multivitamin-mineral supplement to reassure him, but given the way medicine is practiced these days you may have to take the test anyway.

If you have health problems and you are following a nutritionally sound vegetarian diet, it is not likely your diet is the cause, but your doctor may suggest that you need to eat meat. It's worth asking exactly why he or she thinks that meat might help, and doing some research of your own into your condition. You may wish to see a dietitian if you think that your diet is causing your condition, since there may be simple changes that you can make to improve the nutritional quality of your diet, or you may discover that you have a sensitivity to a particular food. It would be a shame to add meat or other animal products back into your diet without very careful research, since there are so many health benefits to a vegetarian diet, and there are many dietary changes that you can make without resorting to meat.

If your doctor is very unsupportive of your diet choice and doesn't respond well to discussing the issues, it may be easier to change doctors than to argue every time you go to visit. Ask friends, especially vegetarian friends, for a recommendation, and find a more supportive doctor. But whatever you do, don't just stop going to the doctor. While the front line doctors still may not have gotten the word on vegetarian diets, the accomplishments of medical science are long and impressive, and visiting a good doctor is usually the best way to get the health care you need.

CHAPTER 10

Eating in Restaurants

What choices do I have when I eat in restaurants?

These days, it's getting easier and easier to eat wholesome vegetarian food in restaurants. Vegetarian restaurants obviously offer the most choices, but you'll also find plenty of good vegetarian food at ethnic restaurants, such as Mexican, Italian, Indian, Chinese, and Thai restaurants, since many of their dishes are focused on vegetables, with beans, lentils, or tofu being the main protein source. Most other restaurants have something available for vegetarians, and even many standard American restaurants offer a veggie burger alternative to the ubiquitous hamburger these days.

Be bold! If nothing on the menu appears to be vegetarian, feel free to ask if something special could be made for you, using ingredients you can see they would have on hand. Many vegetarians have tried this with great success, and very often the chef has appreciated the challenge and the chance to be more creative.

Do your part for the next guy. The more people ask for vegetarian dishes, the more restaurants will recognize the need to offer them. For too long, many vegetarians have been timid in this regard, but the restaurant owners we know tell us they actually like receiving these requests because it gives them a better idea of what people really want.

What should I ask for?

American restaurants: Ask what dishes they have for vegetarians. Be sure to tell your server if you'd like to avoid dairy and eggs, too, and feel free to ask them to hold the cheese, bacon, and mayonnaise as necessary, as these are frequently added to salads and burgers and may not be listed on the menu. Veggie burgers may contain dairy, so it's a good idea to check. To make the meal a little healthier, ask if they have whole wheat bread available and ask for a side of steamed vegetables.

Chinese restaurants: Chinese food usually includes a selection of simple stir-fried vegetables and tofu dishes that go well with rice or noodles. However, in most Chinese restaurants, meat-based dishes dominate the menu, so you may need to ask. The food is not usually highly spiced, although Szechuan dishes can be spicy. Some restaurants may also offer fake meats, made from wheat gluten, which are a delicious choice for vegetarians (and meat eaters). Ask if any vegetable dishes are cooked in a meat or fish broth, so that you can avoid those. Eggs are used in many Chinese dishes, especially fried rice, so ask them to leave the egg out if possible. Ask if they have brown rice available to add extra nutrition.

Ethiopian restaurants: Almost every Ethiopian or Pan-African restaurant serves a veggie combo, consisting of a large *injera* (flatbread) with spoonfuls of various mildly spiced vegetable, lentil, and split pea dishes. It comes with extra *injera* on the side, and you use your fingers to break off the bread, scoop up a bite of vegetables or legumes, and eat it—delicious!

Indian restaurants: Indian food is typically quite spicy, but very tasty. You can usually specify mild, medium, or hot spice levels. *Dal* (lentils) and *channa* (chickpeas) form the basis of many good vegetarian dishes. Appetizers such as vegetable *pakoras* and *samosas* are delicious. Avoid dishes with *paneer* (cheese) and ask whether curry sauces contain dairy or whether they use ghee (butter) for cooking. *Naan* bread usually contains dairy, but *roti* (flatbread) is dairy free and usually made from wholegrain flours.

Italian restaurants: Dishes such as pasta primavera, pasta marinara, and vegetable pizzas are easy options. Italian dishes often contain cheese, but it's worth asking which dishes can be made without dairy, as the chef may be able to make simple substitutions.

Japanese restaurants: Japanese food features a good deal of fish, but there are usually vegetarian options available. Vegetarian sushi, vegetarian tempura, edamame (fresh soybeans), and soybean curd (tofu) are usually available. Miso (soybean paste) is a tasty soup choice. Plain udon or soba noodle dishes, such as yakisoba, flavored with shoyu (soy sauce), are also an option.

Mexican restaurants: Bean burritos, veggie fajitas, and veggie tacos are good bets. Stress that you are vegetarian and ensure that the beans and rice have not been cooked in animal fat or chicken broth. Whole beans can be a safer bet than refried beans if you're not sure. Ask them to hold the cheese, which is added to most dishes, and ask whether their guacamole is made with dairy.

Middle-Eastern restaurants: Falafel (chickpea patties) and hummus (chickpea and tahini dip) are favorites, but grilled eggplant, couscous, dolmades (rice, pine nuts, and spices wrapped in grape leaves), and various salads are usually available. Yogurt is the only dairy product likely to be used, so you can ask them to hold that.

Thai restaurants: Thai dishes use delicious curried sauces and peanut sauce as staples. Many Thai restaurants offer a choice of meat or tofu with any dish, and they often have a separate vegetarian menu. Thai and Chinese restaurants don't use dairy, which makes choosing your meal easier. Fresh tofu is better for you than fried tofu, but both are tasty. Ask if any dishes are cooked in fish sauce, if they don't have a separate vegetarian menu. Eggs may be included in fried rice dishes, so ask them to leave out the egg. Brown rice is often available if you ask.

Vietnamese restaurants: Vietnamese food is similar to Thai food, although peanut sauce is not so common. Often Vietnamese restaurants offer fake meats, so you may be given a vegetarian menu that lists beef-, chicken-, and fish-style dishes. They are all made from wheat gluten and soy and taste very similar to the real meat, although they are 100 percent vegetarian. Other Vietnamese restaurants can be very meat-based, and have very few options for a vegetarian, so it's worth reading the menu carefully before you go in.

Which chain restaurants can I eat in?

Many popular chain restaurants have vegetarian options available. While we don't recommend eating fast food on a regular basis, it is sometimes necessary when you're out and about with limited choices available to you. Here's a list of some of the most readily available outlets in the United States that have choices for vegetarians. There are many restaurant chains in the United States, so this is just a small selection of those available. Thanks to the Vegetarian Resource Group for researching the best options available across the United States:

American:

Burger King: If you have to have a burger, try the BK Veggie Burger. Hold the mayo.

Fresh Choice: You can choose from lots of soups, salads, baked potatoes, and rice and pasta dishes at this salad bar–style restaurant.

Pizza restaurants: Choose a pizza with lots of veggies, ask for extra tomato sauce, and hold the cheese. Some pizza crust ingredients include milk or cheese, so be sure to ask if that's important to you.

Souplantation and Sweet Tomatoes: Choose from lots of soups, salads, and pasta dishes, all clearly labeled as to whether they are vegetarian or vegan.

Subway: Ask for a grilled veggie patty (they are usually available, even if not listed on menu) on a whole wheat sub.

Wendy's: Try a baked potato with broccoli. Hold the sour cream, cheese, and bacon bits.

Mexican:

Chipotle: Try the black bean taco, the fajita burrito, or vegetarian black bean burrito.

Qdoba's Mexican Grill: Try the grilled vegetable burrito, vegetable taco, or salad.

Moe's Southwestern Grill: A vegetarian burrito or taco makes a good choice, or you can replace any meat dish with tofu.

Taco Bell: Try the fresco bean burrito

Taco Del Mar: Specify your own burrito ingredients, including black, pinto, and refried beans (which are not cooked in lard), guacamole (dairy free), rice, salad, and salsa.

Taco Time: Try the veggie burrito or the veggie soft taco. Hold the sour cream and cheese.

Asian:

Noodles & Company: You can choose from noodle dishes, soups, and salads made fresh to order, with many vegetarian options.

Pei Wei Asian Diner: They offer several vegetarian dishes, all clearly labeled, when you choose the dish with vegetables and tofu.

PF Chang's: They have five vegetarian dishes, all clearly labeled. Tofu can be substituted for meat in other dishes, although 40 percent of nonvegetarian dishes are prepared with chicken stock.

CHAPTER 11

Eating at Home

What easy foods can I prepare for myself?

There are many simple vegetarian meals that you can buy in the grocery store and eat almost straight from the container. Others may need heating in a microwave or on the stovetop. In this chapter you'll find plenty of ideas for meals and snacks and will get the lowdown on which ingredients to shop for and why they're great to keep on hand. Chapter 12 gives information about some basic vegetarian staples like tofu, lentils, and vegetables, as well as how to make ingredient substitutions that can transform animal-based meals into vegetarian ones. Chapter 13 is full of simple, basic instructions to get you started, and easy, delicious recipes to enable you to put together complete meals in no time.

But if you're looking for a bit of sophistication, and if you feel ready to attempt more challenging recipes than those included in this book, then you're ready to look for a good cookbook and start being more adventurous. See the Resources section (page 167) for a list of excellent cookbooks.

What can I eat for breakfast?

Don't skip breakfast! Breakfast is an important meal to get your day started right. Eating a decent breakfast every morning can help you maintain a consistent weight. There are many quick and easy, healthful choices available:

Fruit. Fresh fruit, such as oranges, apples, bananas, grapes, or watermelon, is always a good choice. You can combine fresh and frozen fruit with a nondairy milk of your choice into a smoothie for a delicious way to start the day. Try the Protein-Powered Fruit Smoothie (page 130).

Cereal. Choose a natural cereal, made with whole grains for plenty of fiber. Look for brands with as little added sugar as possible and avoid artificial colors and flavors. As for what to pour on your cereal, try various brands of soy, almond, or rice milk until you find one you like. You can even experiment with fruit juice or nondairy yogurt on your cereal for a change.

Bagels. Whole-grain bagels are the healthiest choice. You can buy several fresh bagels at once, slice them, and keep them in a plastic bag in the freezer until you need them. When you're ready to eat one, defrost it in the microwave. Spread it with a nondairy cream cheese that doesn't include hydrogenated fats.

Bread. Choose a natural whole-grain bread. If it's already sliced, you can keep it in a zipper-lock plastic bag in the freezer and just take out slices as you need them. The frozen bread can go directly into a toaster or you can microwave it for fifteen seconds to thaw it out. Top it with nonhydrogenated vegan margarine and cinnamon sugar or jam. Choose a natural brand of jam that lists fruit or fruit purée as the first ingredient. Jelly is usually made from fruit juice, so it has less nutritional value.

Hot breakfasts. When you have a little more time to cook, try whole wheat toaster waffles or pancakes with real maple syrup or a fruit sauce. Tofu scramble with hash browns and veggie sausage or veggie bacon makes a great Sunday brunch. Also try Aunt Amanda's Pancakes (page 132), Tofulicious Scramble (page 133), and Red Potato Vampire Hash Browns (page 134).

What can I eat for lunch?

Lunch is easy. If you want to be sure you have a tasty lunch, it's best to bring your own because many school or office cafeterias have limited vegetarian choices. Many grocery stores have a deli section where you can pick up a salad, hot soup, and a roll to eat for lunch. Check out their sandwich selections, too. If your local supermarket is not very veg-friendly, ask the deli manager for suggestions. If enough people ask, they'll get the idea that more vegetarian options are needed.

Here's a list of easy ideas for lunch, some of which you could pack and bring with you to school or the office, especially if you have access to a microwave to heat your lunch.

Sandwiches. Build your sandwich on a whole-grain foundation. In addition to conventional sliced bread, you can choose pita bread, wraps, tortillas, bagels, or flatbread. Protein-rich filling choices include hummus (a Middle Eastern dip), falafel (spicy chickpea patties), peanut butter and other nut butters, imitation sliced deli meats, nondairy cheese, and sliced baked tofu. Add flavor and nutrition with romaine lettuce, baby spinach leaves, roasted red peppers, zucchini, or other veggies. If you're using pocket bread, consider fillings like coleslaw, beans, and rice. Don't forget the vegan mayonnaise and nonhydrogenated vegan margarine.

Soups and chili. Individual vegetarian soup pots are quick and convenient; just add boiling water and stir. Look for natural brands of canned vegetarian soups and chili. Transfer the soup into a microwave-safe container with a lid and heat it up at school or the office.

Other hot lunches. Premade veggie burritos, wraps, or a slice of quiche (see Kiss-the-Cook Mushroom Quiche, page 144) will reheat nicely.

What can I eat for snacks?

How often have you been saved by a good snack? Here are some snack suggestions. Many of the ideas for breakfast (on page 105) or lunch (on page 106) also make great snacks.

Fruit. The simplest and most nutritious snack choice is fresh fruit. Bananas, apples, oranges, pears, peaches, nectarines, and plums are readily available at the supermarket and easy to carry with you. If you buy melon, such as watermelon, honeydew, or cantaloupe, cut it up and store it in the fridge so it will be ready to eat when the mood strikes you. Grapes, strawberries, and other fresh berries also make good snacks.

Dips. Dips offer good nutrition when they combine whole grains or beans with vegetables. Salsa with whole-grain tortilla chips, hummus with baby carrots, and guacamole or baba ghanouj (eggplant dip) with whole wheat pita chips are just a few possibilities.

Dried fruit and nuts. Eaten in small quantities, nuts and dried fruit can give you a quick energy boost. Good nut choices include cashews, almonds, walnuts, and pistachios. Raisins, dried cranberries, and dried apple slices are all excellent fruit options. Combine dried fruit and nuts to make trail mix, or buy ready-mixed bags. Just make sure to avoid those packed with candy.

Soy or coconut yogurt. Individual cups of yogurt made from soymilk or coconut milk are great when you want a cool, creamy snack.

Nutrition bars. Look for bars with a short list of recognizable ingredients; stay away from those that contain high fructose corn syrup or artificial flavors or colors.

Muffins, cakes, and cookies. Baked goods can be a good choice if you make your own using natural ingredients. See the recipes for Pumpkin Patch Spice Muffins (page 135) and Wild Oatmeal Chocolate Chip Cookies (page 165). Avoid store-bought baked goods that include eggs, dairy, and excess sugar.

What can I eat for dinner?

Polish the day off right with a great dinner. The easiest way to start coming up with dinner ideas is to substitute a prepared meat substitute for the meat in a dish you would usually eat. You can also substitute soymilk and vegan cheese for any dairy ingredients, and use ground flaxseeds or tofu to replace egg ingredients in some recipes. See page 123 for how to replace eggs effectively.

Broaden your horizons. You're off to a good start, but after a while you should aim to widen the variety of options available to you, and look for ways to base more of your meals around vegetables. Here is a list of easy meal suggestions. Recipes for most of these suggestions are included in chapter 13. You can also adapt many of the lunch ideas listed above into dinner ideas.

Potato-based meals. A baked potato loaded with nutritious toppings, such as baked beans, vegetarian chili, peas, corn, or vegan cheese, makes a satisfying meal. Vegan sour cream and veggie bacon bits provide the finishing touch. Serve mashed potatoes with grilled veggie sausages or other meat substitutes, plus a fresh steamed vegetable or two, such as broccoli, carrots, green beans, or peas. Or combine boiled potatoes with carrots, peas, and pasta and cover with cheeze sauce to make a hot pot (see page 145).

Pasta-based meals. Vegetarian lasagne made with tofu and spinach is an impressive meal to serve your family. Give marinara sauce a nutritional boost by adding vegetables and beans before ladling it over pasta. Mac 'n Cheeze (page 143) recreates an old favorite, vegan style. Pesto sauce makes a nice change of pace or, for a more exotic touch, try spaghetti with peanut sauce (see Marco Polo Peanut Butter Pasta, page 149). Don't forget to serve a salad or steamed veggies on the side.

Bread-based meals. Sandwiches aren't just for lunch; fold some vegetarian chili into a burrito, wrap, or tortilla, or try sloppy joes made with tempeh. Serve them with a salad for some extra nutrition and crunch.

Rice-based meals. Rice is the foundation of many of the world's great meals. The possibilities are endless when it comes to stir-fries with tofu and vegetables. Indian and Thai curries and Italian risotto also provide plenty of delicious ways to combine rice and vegetables (note that quinoa substitutes well for rice in any meal).

What's for dessert?

Desserts can be good for you! The most healthful dessert is a piece of fresh fruit or a serving of fruit salad (page 125). But you'll be pleased to know that dark chocolate (dairy free) is actually very good for you in moderation. However, most commercial cakes, cookies, and puddings use dairy products, eggs, and lots of sugar, so it's better to skip those or make your own. Fruit sorbet and dairy-free ice cream are available in most grocery stores; try them topped with a sprinkle of toasted wheat germ. Here are a few more simple suggestions:

> Chocolate Bonbons (page 164)
> Creamy Chocolate Dream Pudding (page 161)
> Grandma's Apple Crisp (page 162)
> Passion for Pumpkin Pie (page 163)
> Wild Oatmeal Chocolate Chip Cookies (page 165)

What foods should I keep available?

Here's kitchen management 101! As you try new recipes and become familiar with new foods, the foods that you keep available at home will change. Remember that fresh fruits and vegetables are best eaten within a week, so don't buy more than you can eat. Instead, try to buy different ones each week depending on what's in season, to add variety to your diet. Frozen vegetables and berries are usually cheaper than fresh, especially in the winter, and they are also more convenient to use, so these are good products to have on hand, especially for soups, stews, and smoothies. Some foods, such as tomatoes, pumpkin, and most types of beans, are much more convenient from a can, with very little lost nutritionally.

What should I include in my shopping list?

Don't get lost in the store. Make a list to find your way through. Use the following guidelines as a starting point for your shopping list. You may find that your local grocery store doesn't carry all the items listed here, but it will probably carry most of them, especially if it has a natural foods section. Try a natural food store, or a more specialized grocery store, to buy any items you can't buy in your regular store.

To determine whether an item is natural or not, look at the ingredient list. If the list is short and you recognize the names of the ingredients, then it's a pretty natural product. If the list of ingredients requires a PhD in chemistry to decipher then it's probably not such a great choice.

Baking Supplies

Baking powder and baking soda. Both baking powder and baking soda are leavenings that are used to make baked goods rise, but they work in different ways, so you will need to buy both. When buying baking powder, choose an aluminum-free brand.

Chocolate chips. Nondairy chocolate chips are great in small amounts as a snack, added to cookies, or melted on strawberries, apple slices, or nondairy ice cream.

Cocoa powder. Cocoa powder can be natural or dutch processed. Dutch-processed cocoa powder is less acidic than natural cocoa, but they can usually be used interchangeably.

Nutritional yeast. Nutritional yeast are powdery yellow flakes that have a savory flavor and are useful for making cheeze sauces.

Sweeteners. Even natural sweeteners are still basically sugar, so they are high in calories and should be used sparingly.
> agave nectar: Agave nectar comes from a cactus plant. It is relatively flavorless and good for sweetening beverages as well as baked goods.
> brown rice syrup: Thick and sticky, brown rice syrup has a slight butterscotch flavor and is used in baking.
> evaporated cane juice: Although it has "juice" in its name, evaporated cane juice is a granulated sweetener like sugar, but less refined.
> maple syrup: Real maple syrup is expensive but much more wholesome than pancake syrup, which is artificially flavored corn syrup.

Vanilla extract. Typically sold in liquid form, with alcohol to retain freshness, pure vanilla extract is more expensive but has a much better taste than artificial vanilla flavoring.

Whole wheat pastry flour. More nutritious than plain white flour, whole wheat pastry flour is good for baking. It has a softer texture than regular whole wheat flour.

Beverages

Fruit juice. Fruit juice is better for you than soda, but it does contain a lot of calories and sugar, so don't drink excessive amounts. Try mixing fruit juice with seltzer or plain water. When buying juice, look for 100 percent juice with no sugar added. Orange juice with added calcium is also a good choice.

Soymilk and other milk alternatives. If you like to drink milk, then switch to one of these, but again the calories can add up if you drink large quantities. Try to stick to plain, unsweetened varieties.

Tea. Green and black tea both contain antioxidants and are available decaffeinated. Fruit-flavored teas are also tasty and a great way to have a hot drink without adding calories.

Water. The best drink you can put in your body is plain old water. There's no need to buy bottled water; tap water is fine in most American cities. You can filter it if you are worried about the taste or any toxic chemicals that could be in it.

Canned and jarred goods

Beans. Canned beans are more expensive than dried but much more convenient. Keep a few varieties on hand: black beans and chickpeas, for example, plus prepared items, such as refried beans, vegetarian baked beans, and vegetarian chili.

Coconut milk. Coconut milk is unsweetened and available in a full-fat version and a "lite," or reduced-fat version. It is essential for many Thai curries and soups. Don't confuse coconut milk with cream of coconut, a thick, sweetened product.

Fruit. Canned peaches and pineapple taste great with nondairy vanilla ice cream or added to salad. Look for canned fruit packed in natural juices, not heavy syrup.

Lemon and lime juices. Bottled lemon and lime juices can be used in place of freshly squeezed juice in salad dressings and other recipes when you don't have the fresh fruit available. Choose pure juice rather than a product containing lemon or lime oil, and store it in the refrigerator.

Miso. Miso is made from soybeans and sometimes other beans and grains. It can be added to soups or used to make broth.

Nut butters. Peanut butter is the most readily available, but others such as almond, soynut, or sunflower butters are good too. Choose a natural brand without sugar and stabilizers. You'll need to stir in the oil and then keep it refrigerated.

Oils and vinegars.

> ➢ balsamic vinegar: Thick and slightly sweet, balsamic vinegar is used for marinades and salad dressings.
> ➢ brown rice vinegar: Brown rice vinegar adds zing to homemade Asian sauces.
> ➢ canola oil: Neutral-tasting canola oil is a good all-purpose oil for baking and cooking.
> ➢ flaxseed oil: Flaxseed oil is a very good source of beneficial omega-3 fatty acids. It should not be heated; use it in salad dressings or toss it with cooked pasta.
> ➢ olive oil: Extra-virgin olive oil is best for salad dressings (it breaks down when heated). Regular olive oil is good for cooking.
> ➢ sesame oil: Untoasted sesame oil can be used in cooking. Toasted sesame oil has a distinctive smoky flavor and is used for dressings or added to dishes at the end of cooking.

Pumpkin. Canned pumpkin is just as nutritious as fresh pumpkin and is great to keep on hand for making muffins, quick bread, and pie.

Soy sauce. Regular soy sauce, made with wheat, is also called shoyu. Tamari is a type of soy sauce made without wheat. Whichever you buy, look for a low-sodium brand.

Tahini. Tahini is a savory butter made from sesame seeds, used in Middle Eastern dishes such as hummus and baba ghanouj.

Tomatoes. Diced tomatoes are a must-have for your pantry year-round to use in soups, stews, and curries. Look for brands with no salt added.

Dried beans, grains, and other staples

Lentils. It's a good idea to have both red and brown lentils on hand. Red lentils break down to a porridgelike consistency when cooked, while brown lentils retain their shape.

Oats. Choose rolled oats to serve for a hot breakfast and quick-cooking oats for cookies and apple crisp.

Nuts and seeds. Because nuts and seeds are high in oil, it is important that they be fresh. Buy from a store that sells them quickly, and store them in the refrigerator. Whole nuts stay fresh longer than chopped nuts.

> - almonds: Almonds are high in protein, fiber, and vitamin E.
> - cashews: Cashews taste great in Asian stir-fries.
> - flaxseeds: Flaxseeds can be ground and used to replace eggs in baked goods.
> - peanuts: Buy peanuts in the shell for snacking.
> - pumpkin seeds: Also called pepitas, pumpkin seeds can be eaten as a snack or added to baked goods.
> - sunflower seeds: Sunflower seeds add crunch and nutrition to salads.
> - walnuts: Walnuts are high in polyunsaturated fats, including omega-3 fatty acids.

Pasta. Whole wheat and whole-grain pasta are available in a variety of shapes.

Quinoa. Quinoa is a great high-protein grain to add to your diet.

Rice. Brown rice is healthiest because it includes the bran. Choose long or short grain, whichever you prefer.

Textured Soy Protein (TSP). TSP is very versatile and adds protein to stews and casseroles.

Veggie bacon crumbles. Veggie bacon crumbles add flavor and crunch to salads.

Wheat germ. Buy toasted wheat germ in a jar or untoasted wheat germ in bulk, to sprinkle on salads and desserts for extra nutrition.

Frozen foods

Meat alternatives. Frozen meat alternatives include veggie burgers, veggie sausages, "meatballs," and "chicken" nuggets. They make getting a meal on the table quick and easy.

Sorbet and nondairy ice cream. Fruity sorbet and creamy nondairy ice cream make a good summer dessert or snack. Nondairy frozen desserts may be based on fruit, soymilk, or rice milk.

Vegetables. Keep a few bags of frozen vegetables on hand for times when you run out of fresh vegetables or want a quick way to add extra nutrients to a meal. Good choices include peas, corn, spinach, and mixed vegetables.

Veggie burritos and wraps. Frozen veggie burritos, wraps, and other frozen meals can kept on hand for when you're just too busy to cook.

Herbs and spices

Herbs. Dried herbs add variety and interest to meals. Commonly used herbs include basil, oregano, and thyme. Buy only as much as you can use in six months or so.

Pepper. Black pepper is available ground or as whole peppercorns. Freshly ground pepper is more pungent than the preground variety.

Salt. Natural sea salt contains many other minerals in addition to sodium chloride, so it's better for you than table salt.

Spices. Many spices, such as cinnamon, cloves, and ginger, can be used both for baking desserts and cooking savory dishes. Spices, such as cumin, coriander, and turmeric, and spice blends, like chili powder, are handy to have in your pantry for making curries.

Prepared foods

Bread. Look for whole-grain sliced bread and store it in a plastic bag in the freezer, so that you always have fresh bread available. Also good to have on hand (and easily stored in the freezer) are whole-grain pita pockets, hamburger and hot dog buns, bagels, and pizza crusts.

Cereal. Choose natural whole-grain cereal and make sure it has plenty of fiber.

Chocolate sauce. Natural chocolate sauce is a treat poured over nondairy ice cream or used as a dip for strawberries and bananas.

Condiments. Ketchup and mustard are a must on veggie burgers and hot dogs. Find natural brands if you can, to avoid added sugar and chemicals. Dijon mustard is spicier than yellow mustard and adds a kick to salad dressings and other recipes.

Curry paste. Thai curry pastes can be used with coconut milk to create a variety of flavors.

Curry sauce. Look for Indian curries without dairy ingredients. Thai curry sauces are based on coconut milk so there's no need to worry about dairy in those.

Falafel. Dried falafel mix is a convenient way to make chickpea patties quickly.

Salad dressings. Buy a few different salad dressings to add variety to your daily salad. Choose natural dressings without dairy ingredients.

Salsa. In addition to dipping chips into salsa, you can use it to top beans, spread on enchiladas, and spoon onto tacos.

Soup. Look for low-salt natural soups and chili without lots of additives. Dried individual soup pots, canned soups, and aseptically packaged soups are all good choices that will keep well until you need them.

Tomato sauce. Basic tomato sauce can be dressed up with herbs and used for pizza or pasta.

Vegetable broth. You can buy broth in aseptic containers but powder, paste, or cubes are cheaper; just add hot water.

Vegan mayonnaise. Vegan mayonnaise is made with tofu instead of eggs, and is very useful for sandwiches and coleslaw.

Produce

Fruit. Buy lots of fruit, then wash it when you get home and have it ready to eat. That way you'll be more likely to choose fruit for a quick and wholesome snack. Choose whichever fruits are your favorites to eat fresh. It's cheaper to buy fruit in season, so check with the produce manager at your local store to find the best seasons for your favorite fruits.

> apples: Apples are good for both snacking and baking. Try different varieties to see which ones you like best.

> bananas: Fresh bananas are useful for smoothies. Save ripe ones to make bread and muffins, or peel them and put them in zipper-lock plastic bags in the freezer for use in smoothies later.

> berries: Fresh berries add color and flavor to breakfast cereal, hot or cold. Check carefully to make sure they are free of mold.

> citrus fruits: Grapefruit, lemons, limes, and oranges are good to keep on hand for juicing as well as snacking.

> grapes: Red or green grapes make great snacks. They can also be frozen for a refreshing, cold treat.

> soft fruits: Mangos, nectarines, peaches, pears, and plums are delicious fresh and can be used in smoothies once they're past their prime.

Vegetables. Choose a variety of vegetables that includes root vegetables, leafy greens, and another vegetable, such as broccoli or mushrooms, each week, plus whatever salad items you can eat.

➤ broccoli and cauliflower: Related cruciferous vegetables, broccoli and cauliflower are both versatile and nutritious. The head should be firm and free of yellow spots or blemishes.

➤ cabbage: Green cabbage and purple cabbage are good for coleslaw and stir-fries. You can also find Asian cabbage, such as napa and bok choy.

➤ eggplants: Eggplants come in a variety of colors and sizes but the large purple variety is the most common. Fresh eggplant has tight, shiny skin.

➤ ginger: Although it's not a vegetable, you'll find fresh ginger in the produce section with the vegetables. It comes in large pieces but you can break off the amount that you need. Ginger keeps well in the freezer in a sealed plastic bag and is also easier to grate when frozen.

➤ greens: Collards and kale are sturdy, long-cooking greens; spinach and swiss chard are more tender. Pre-washed bags of greens are quick and easy to use.

➤ mushrooms: The most commonly available mushrooms include cremini, portobello, shiitake, and white mushrooms. Cremini (small brown) and regular white mushrooms are similar and can be used interchangeably in recipes. Shiitake mushrooms have a chewy texture. Portobello mushrooms are very large, and can be marinated and grilled whole and served like a burger.

➤ okra: Okra is a fuzzy, green vegetable popular in Indian, Caribbean, and Southern U.S. cuisines. It's also known as *bhindi*, gumbo, and lady's fingers. When buying fresh okra, choose ones that are small, firm, and dry.

➤ onions and garlic: Onions and garlic store well in a cool, dry place. They are essential for many stews and curries.

➤ root vegetables: Root vegetables, such as carrots, parsnips, potatoes, sweet potatoes, and yams, should be firm and free of blemishes.

➤ salad vegetables: In addition to lettuce, choose avocados, bell peppers, cucumbers, and tomatoes to give your salad color and flavor.

➤ squash: Choose small to medium summer squash and zucchini for the best flavor. Winter squash, such as butternut, delicata, and spaghetti squash, should be heavy for its size, with no soft spots.

Refrigerated foods

Cheese alternatives. Choose a nondairy, nonhydrogenated (also known as trans fat-free) margarine to replace butter. Nondairy cream cheese and cheese slices are great to keep on hand to go with bagels and sandwiches.

Dips and spreads. Prepared hummus, guacamole, salsa, and other dips and spreads can be used as the basis of a nutritious snack or light meal.

Meat alternatives. Great for making a quick sandwich, meat alternatives such as deli-style slices, hot dogs, and sausages are sometimes found in the refrigerated section of the produce aisle.

Milk alternatives. Soymilk, almond milk, and rice milk may be in the refrigerated section or in aseptic packs in the dry goods section. They should be refrigerated after opening.

Pesto. Prepared pesto is an easy topping for pasta. Because most brands contain dairy products, be sure to check the ingredient list.

Pie crust. Premade whole wheat pie crusts enable you to cook pies and quiches quickly; look for a brand made without butter.

Seitan. Seitan is a meat substitute made from wheat gluten and is sold plain or flavored.

Soy yogurt. Small cups of soy yogurt are great to have on hand as a snack, breakfast, or even dessert.

Tempeh. Tempeh is made from fermented soybeans and sometimes other grains. It may be stored in the refrigerator or freezer.

Tofu. Choose regular tofu for stir-fries and scrambles. Silken tofu is best for smoothies and puddings. Marinated baked tofu can be used in salads and sandwiches straight from the package. Check the "sell-by" date and keep unused tofu in the refrigerator.

CHAPTER 12

Ingredient Basics

What can I use in place of meat in my everyday meals?

Start with soy! Soybean products, such as tofu, tempeh, and textured vegetable protein, are popular with new vegetarians because they can replace meat in easy meals like stir-fries and chili. Other beans (and foods made from beans, such as hummus and falafel) can be used to make sandwiches, salads, and stews more nutritious. Seitan, a wheat product, can be made to look and taste like meat. Nuts, seeds, and nut butters are also valuable sources of protein. Prepared meat alternatives, such as burgers, nuggets, pepperoni, sausages, or veggie bacon, are generally made from wheat gluten or soy (or both), as they are very high in protein, complex carbohydrates, fiber, and other nutrients.

What is tofu?

Tofu is made from soybeans, and is a very good source of protein. There are two main types—regular tofu and silken tofu. Regular tofu is sold as a white cake, usually floating in water. Fresh tofu has no smell and has a very mild flavor. It may be labeled soft, firm, or extra firm, which refers to the amount of water absorbed into the tofu. This type of tofu is good as a meat substitute when marinated. After draining the water from the package and patting the tofu dry, you can cut it into cubes or crumble it and add it to a variety of dishes, such as stir-fries, curries, stews, and scrambles. Tofu must be stored in the refrigerator and used before its "sell by" date. If you use part of a package, store the remaining tofu in a container of water in the refrigerator. The texture of tofu changes considerably if you freeze it, which enables it to absorb more marinade flavor. You can also buy pre-marinated tofu, which comes in a variety of flavors and is ready to eat or to add to stir-fries. Baked marinated tofu has a particularly firm texture and can be sliced and used in sandwiches, or cubed and added to salads straight from the package.

Silken tofu has a much creamier texture, and is more useful in dishes with a creamy consistency, such as quiches, puddings, or smoothies. It is too soft to be cubed or crumbled. It is usually sold in an aseptic package and can be stored at room temperature for several months. You can put it in the refrigerator the day before using it, if you plan to use it in a chilled item such as a smoothie.

What is tempeh?

Tempeh is made by fermenting soybeans and then pressing them into a cake form. It is high in protein, has a firm texture, and makes a great substitute for meat. It has a nutty flavor of its own but absorbs other flavors well and takes well to marinades. Marinated tempeh can be crumbled to make sloppy joes or left in large pieces and grilled to make a tasty burger substitute. It is also sliced very thin to make a bacon substitute. Tempeh keeps well in the refrigerator for a couple of weeks and longer in the freezer; you can defrost it quickly in the microwave when you're ready to use it.

What is textured soy protein?

Textured soy protein, or TSP, is made from soybean flour that has been cooked and dried, and is sold as flakes or crumbles. Like tofu, it takes on the flavor of whatever sauce you cook it in. You can add TSP to soups and stews to add protein or use it in spaghetti sauce to make a dish similar to sloppy joes. Because it is dried, TSP can be stored at room temperature.

What is seitan?

Seitan is made from wheat gluten and has a chewy texture somewhat like chicken. It is the main ingredient in the realistic fake meats served at some vegetarian restaurants. At the supermarket, seitan is sold in the refrigerated section. It comes in irregular chunks, which can be sliced or left whole. Seitan is a good addition to stews and it can also be marinated, then grilled or roasted.

What types of beans are there?

Beans come in a huge array of colors, sizes, and flavors. The most commonly available beans include adzuki beans, black (or turtle) beans, black-eyed peas, cannellini, chickpeas (or garbanzo beans), great northern beans, kidney beans, lima (or butter) beans, pinto beans, and red beans. All are high in protein, fiber, and other nutrients, and so they make a good addition to your diet. If you are new to eating beans, start by eating small quantities so that your body can get used to the additional fiber, which may cause gas. Some beans, such as kidney beans and black-eyed peas, are less digestible and cause more gas than others, so bear that in mind when choosing which beans to try first.

Dried beans can take an hour or two to cook, depending on the type and whether they have been soaked. Canned beans are a lot quicker to use because they are already cooked. Open the can, drain off the liquid, and fill up the can with fresh water to rinse the beans. Drain off the rinse water and then add the beans to your recipe.

What is special about lentils?

Lentils deserve more respect. Lentils, and their close relatives, split peas, are more digestible than beans and take less time to cook, so it doesn't save a lot of time to use canned lentils. There are several different varieties of lentils to choose from, especially if you go to an Indian grocery, where they're known as *dal*. The most common ones are red lentils and brown lentils. Red lentils are particularly high in iron. They cook quickly and collapse into a yellow colored paste that can be served plain or combined with vegetables and spices to make a curry (see Benny Bengali's Indian Curry, page 156). Brown lentils hold their shape when cooked, and are tasty in soups and salads.

What is hummus?

This Middle Eastern spread and dip is a winner. It is made from chickpeas and tahini (sesame seed butter), with lemon juice and garlic. You can buy it prepared or make your own (see Garlic Lover's Hummus, page 136). It's a tasty dip for vegetable sticks and chips. Hummus can also be used as a spread in sandwiches.

What is falafel?

You're going to love falafel. Falafel is a mixture of chickpeas and spices that is formed into small patties, then cooked and tucked into pita bread pockets. You can easily make your falafel using a packaged mix. Cooked falafel will keep in the refrigerator for a few days. Serve with a simple tahini dip (see Tasty Tahini Sauce, page 138).

Which nuts and seeds are good to eat?

Nuts are a very valuable addition to your diet—they're high in protein and fiber and while they contain a lot of fat, it is the good, unsaturated kind. The most popular nuts are almonds, brazil nuts, cashew nuts, coconut, hazelnuts, macadamia nuts, peanuts (technically legumes but considered nuts), pecans, pine nuts, pistachios, and walnuts. Walnuts are particularly nutritious. All nuts make a great snack on their own or added to trail mix, and they can be sprinkled on salads, made into a nut roast (like a vegetarian meatloaf), added to baked goods, and ground into butters or sauces. Just don't overdo eating nuts if you're watching your weight, because they are quite high in calories—a handful or two every couple of days does it.

Seeds are not just for the birds; they add crunch and extra nutrition to your diet. Poppy, pumpkin, sesame, and sunflower seeds are the most commonly available. Sprinkle them, raw or toasted, on salads or on breads and muffins before baking them.

Which nut butters can I use?

Peanut butter is the most popular nut butter and comes in many styles—crunchy, creamy, salted, unsalted, natural, or sweetened. Pure peanut butter is made by simply grinding up peanuts, although many commercial brands include salt, sweeteners, and oils, such as palm oil, to stabilize the peanut butter and prevent it from separating. Peanut butter is the main ingredient in a Thai peanut sauce which adds flavor and nutrition to many a Thai recipe.

Go beyond peanut butter. Almonds and cashews are also ground into butter, which can be used the same way as peanut butter, in sandwiches, cookies, and sauces. Tahini is butter made from ground sesame seeds and is used in hummus as well as other spreads and sauces.

What can I use to replace cow's milk?

Save the cow's milk for the calves. There are many nondairy milks available these days. Soymilk is the most popular, but almond milk, rice milk, oat milk, hazelnut milk, and hemp milk are available in many natural food stores. When choosing which milk to use, find a flavor you like and compare the nutrients. Most have calcium, and vitamins A and D added. Some have other vitamins and minerals added too. Soymilk has high levels of protein, whereas other milks have less. In most recipes, alternative milks work just as effectively as low-fat cow's milk.

What can I use to replace cheese?

Say "cheeze" instead! Nutritional yeast has a distinctly cheesy flavor. It comes as a yellow powder or flakes, and can be added to a basic sauce to make a good cheeze sauce (see Say Cheeze Sauce, page 143). You can also choose from several brands of soy, rice, or almond cheese available in grated, sliced, or block form. Many of these products use casein, a cows milk protein, to help them melt better, so if you're trying to eliminate all dairy products, you'll need to look carefully at the ingredient list.

What can I use to replace eggs?

Eggs are not essential but they are used in many different ways in recipes, so the choice of replacement has to fit the purpose. To replace scrambled eggs, regular tofu crumbled, with spices added (try the Tofulicious Scramble, page 133) is a good substitute. To replace eggs in baked goods, a tablespoon of ground flaxseeds, a mashed banana, or silken tofu can work well. You'll need to experiment with your favorite recipes to see which works best for you. You can also buy powdered egg replacer, which contains potato starch, to use in some baking recipes.

What are whole grains?

Grains are great! You can buy the most commonly used grains—corn, oats, rice, and wheat—in their unrefined form. Many supermarkets now sell lesser-known and exotic grains, such as amaranth, barley, buckwheat, bulgur, millet, quinoa, rye, spelt, and teff. To understand the difference between a whole grain and a refined grain, think of rice as an example. A grain of rice is mainly starch, with an oil-rich germ, a layer of protective bran, and an inedible hull. Removing just the hull produces brown rice, a whole grain. To produce white rice, the bran and germ are removed as well. Since the bran and the germ contain valuable nutrients including fiber, it is better to eat brown rice whenever possible.

Discover flour power. Whole wheat and other grains are ground into flour, which is used to make bread, cakes, and cookies. Because different grains offer slightly different nutrients, baked goods labeled "whole grain" are better than those labeled "whole wheat," which in turn are better for you than products made from white (refined) flour. Pasta, including spaghetti and couscous, is made with durum wheat flour, but whole-grain pasta is becoming increasingly available. Many people new to healthful eating consume the bulk of the grains in their diet as bread and pasta. The whole-grain versions are nutritious, but it's best to include a variety of grains in your diet, so try expanding the range of grains to include at least rice, corn, and oats. Rice is used in many ethnic meals, so it is easily included in your diet. Cornmeal is used in chips, tortillas, polenta, and cornbread, and many other foods. Look for products that are made with stone-ground cornmeal, which contains more nutrients. Steel-cut oats are mainly used as a hot breakfast, while old-fashioned oats and quick oats can also be used in baked goods. Avoid instant oats, which have been precooked and dried, with flavorings and sweeteners added.

If you're feeling adventurous, try some of the less familiar grains, starting with quinoa. Quinoa (pronounced keen-wah) is particularly high in protein and cooks very quickly, so it is an easy grain to prepare. In its uncooked state it looks like tiny white beads. When cooked, it fluffs up to look like couscous or round rice.

What natural sweeteners can I use?

Natural sweeteners are less refined than white sugar, and so have more nutrients (although they have just as many calories). Examples include agave nectar, brown rice syrup, honey, and maple syrup (not maple-flavored corn syrup). You can also use puréed fruit, such as bananas, or applesauce to provide added sweetness.

Liquid sweeteners work in many recipes, but sometimes you need a granulated sweetener. Evaporated cane juice, which looks like brown sugar but is less refined, can be used like white sugar. A calorie-free alternative to sugar is an herb called stevia. Stevia is much sweeter than sugar and is used in very small amounts.

How can I include more fruits and vegetables in my diet?

Take fruits and veggies seriously—they are an important component of your diet, and most of us don't eat enough of them. The American Cancer Society advises us all to eat at least five servings of fruits and vegetables every day, and many experts suggest that eight to ten servings per day would be optimal. The only way to achieve this is to plan each meal to include several servings of fruits or vegetables.

For breakfast, focus on fruit. A smoothie (see Protein-Powered Fruit Smoothie, page 130) is a great way to get plenty of fruit into your diet, as you can include bananas and whatever fruit you have on hand. Alternatively, a glass of orange juice, and a piece of fruit on the side of whatever else you have for breakfast will get you started on meeting your fruit requirement for the day.

For lunch, try to include a couple of different vegetables with the meal. This can be as simple as tucking some greens, cucumber slices, and red pepper sticks into your sandwich. Choose romaine, red leaf lettuce, or spinach rather than iceberg lettuce, which has little nutritional value. Baby carrots, zucchini, and red pepper sticks are great to dip into hummus or other dips. Coleslaw (see The Great American Coleslaw, page 139) is a delicious option in a pita pocket, and vegetable soups are always a good choice. A piece of fruit makes a great dessert.

For a snack, grab a piece of fruit, a bowl of trail mix with dried fruit, or a handful of baby carrots.

For dinner, choose an entrée that includes plenty of vegetables, and add more if you can. For example, most frozen vegetable pizzas come topped with just a few small pieces of vegetables. If you load a store-bought pizza up with extra vegetables—sliced mushrooms, zucchini, red peppers, peas, and corn kernels—you're adding flavor, as well as nutrition and fiber. In addition to the main course, aim to always have at least one steamed vegetable and a bowl of salad on the side. Good choices for steamed vegetables include kale, collards, chard, green beans, and broccoli, although any vegetable you like is a good choice. Remember that variety is important, so try to vary your choice of vegetables from one day to the next.

How do I make fruit salad?

Any fresh fruit that holds its shape well can be used for a fruit salad. Good choices include apples, bananas, grapes, mandarin orange segments, all types of melons, pears, and strawberries. Make sure to wash the fruit first, cut larger fruit into bite-sized chunks, then gently combine the fruit in a bowl. Prepare the salad as close to eating time as possible because chopped fruit (especially apples, pears, and bananas) browns and spoils quickly. If you need to prepare it in advance, sprinkle a little lemon juice over the salad and toss gently to limit the browning. Refrigerate after preparing to keep it fresh.

How do I prepare vegetables?

The first rule for vegetables is to always wash them under running water before using them. Vegetables are often sold unwrapped, and any number of people may have handled them before you buy them. Here are some tips for preparing the most commonly used vegetables:

Broccoli. Wash the broccoli, then trim the woody end from the stem. Chop the remaining stem into slices and separate the head into individual florets. Broccoli is often simply steamed or added to stir-fries. It tastes best when cooked just until it's tender but retains some bite and the color is still bright green.

Cauliflower. Wash the cauliflower, then cut the whole head in half. Slice the florets from the central stem and discard the stem. Separate the florets into bite-sized pieces. Whether steamed or added to a curry or stew, cauliflower takes about fifteen minutes to become tender.

Eggplants. Rinse or peel the eggplant, then cut it into thick slices before grilling with a little oil, or chop it into cubes to add to stews. Note that eggplant flesh browns quickly once cut, so don't prepare it too far in advance of cooking it. Baba ghanouj is a dip made from grilled eggplant (see Ali Baba's Ghanouj, page 137).

Green beans. Rinse the beans well and then trim both ends. Steam them, covered with a lid, for five minutes on the stovetop or two minutes in the microwave.

Greens. Fresh greens, such as bok choy, chard, collards, kale, lettuce, or spinach, can contain a lot of grit and dirt and must be washed thoroughly; a large bowl of water is ideal for this, as any soil will sink to the bottom. With curly kale, you'll need to use your fingers to rub into every fold to make sure they're clean. Remove any tough stems and chop or tear the leaves into bite-sized pieces.

If serving the greens in a salad, you can shake them dry or spin them in a salad spinner to remove the excess water. Prewashed salad leaves can be used right out of the bag, although it is advisable to give them another quick rinse if you have time.

To cook greens, either steam them with a little water for just a few minutes until tender, or add them directly to a soup or stew. It is better to cook greens for as little time as possible to retain the best nutrients. Bagged frozen spinach can be added to a soup or stew directly where it will defrost in just a few minutes. Spinach frozen in a block must be defrosted in the microwave or in a bowl of hot water before use.

Mushrooms. To prepare mushrooms, rinse them well, rubbing the caps with your thumbs to remove any dirt. Shiitake mushrooms have a tough stem, which should be removed. The stems of white, cremini, and portobello mushrooms can be removed or merely trimmed. Slice, chop, or quarter the mushrooms as needed. To grill portobello mushrooms, remove the stem and marinate them in barbecue sauce before putting them on the grill.

Onions. To prepare an onion, cut off the top and bottom and remove the papery skin. Cut the onion crosswise into slices for onion rings. To dice an onion, first cut it in half from stem to root end. Place each half flat on a chopping board and cut it into slices lengthwise, then crosswise into small pieces.

Root vegetables. Carrots, parsnips, potatoes, sweet potatoes, and yams can either be peeled or scrubbed clean and served with the skin on. The skin contains valuable nutrients, so it's better to leave it on. Remove any bad parts, sprouted roots, or eyes with a knife before cutting. The best ways to cook root vegetables include boiling, roasting, and baking. When you bake a potato or sweet potato, be sure to pierce it in a few places with a fork. This will allow steam to escape and prevent the potato from exploding while it cooks.

Squashes. Summer squash and zucchini have tender skins and seeds, and just need to be rinsed and sliced before cooking. Winter squash, such as acorn, butternut, delicata, pumpkin, and spaghetti squash, must be cut open and the seeds removed. They can then be baked, roasted, steamed, or added to soups or stews. The skin of delicata squash is tender enough to be eaten; for other varieties of winter squash you can remove the peel either before cooking or after.

Tomatoes. Tomatoes can simply be rinsed, then cut into wedges for salads, thick slices for burgers and sandwiches, or chunks for soups and stews. Fresh tomatoes are delicious in salads or inside a burger. They can also be cooked in soups and stews or made into sauce for pizzas and pasta, although it is often easier to use canned tomatoes or a jar of marinara sauce for these purposes.

What are trans fats and why should I avoid them?

Trans fats are bad for you. Also known as partially hydrogenated fats, they used to be a main ingredient in margarines and the main fat in most baked goods and junk foods. Food manufacturers like to use them because they help keep food fresh for a longer time and don't go rancid so easily. However, they've been found to be really bad for our health, and it is now required by U.S. law to list the amount of trans fats in the "nutrition facts" section of product labels. As a result, manufacturers have been cutting back on their use of trans fats quite rapidly, but you should still check the ingredient list of packaged foods and avoid any products that have the words "partially hydrogenated" listed.

What oils and fats should I use?

Use a fresh, simple vegetable oil. Canola oil has a very mild taste and can be heated without being damaged, so it can be used in baked goods and for frying. It is particularly low in saturated fat and higher in omega-3 fatty acids than other oils, which means that it is a good choice. Safflower, sunflower, and corn oils are also useful oils, although they have less omega-3 fats. Just avoid generic vegetable oil, which may include other less nutritious oils.

Many people prefer the taste of extra-virgin olive oil for making salad dressings. This is a good choice, but don't use extra-virgin olive oil for cooking as it breaks down into less nutritious compounds under heat.

If you need a more solid spread for sandwiches or cooking, choose one that is nonhydrogenated and labeled as having no trans fats. It will be much lower in saturated fat than butter and won't have the trans fats found in most margarines. Avoid lard at all costs, as it is made from pork fat.

CHAPTER 13

Recipes

Let's start cooking. Here are some useful recipes to get you started. Some people feel safest sticking precisely to a recipe, while others see recipes as a starting point for experimentation. We have included tips and variations to encourage you to experiment, but you can always stick to the basic ingredients to keep it simple. If you're ready for more variety, there are many good vegetarian cookbooks available. See the Resources section (page 167) for a list of recommendations.

Breakfast

Protein-Powered Fruit Smoothie

Makes 1 serving

THIS SIMPLE FRUIT DRINK tastes great using whatever fruit you have on hand. The tofu adds creaminess as well as protein.

1 fresh or frozen banana, sliced or broken into pieces
1/2 cup fresh or frozen fruit (such as blueberries or strawberries)
1/2 cup soymilk, almond milk, or orange juice
1/4 cup silken tofu (optional)
Water or ice cubes, as needed

Put all the ingredients in a blender and process until smooth. Add water or ice cubes to achieve the desired consistency.

Tips:

➢ To freeze bananas, peel them, then place them in a heavy-duty zipper-lock plastic bag, squeezing out as much air as possible. Stored in the bag in the freezer, they will keep for about 2 weeks.

➢ Always use one frozen fruit, to chill the smoothie.

➢ Although a blender will provide the best results, you can use a food processor for this recipe. Process the banana and frozen fruit first, until smooth. Then add the remaining ingredients and process again to achieve the desired consistency.

Old-Fashioned Oatmeal

Makes 4 servings

THICK-CUT ROLLED OATS make a hearty, stick-to-your-ribs breakfast; they're in a different league from the instant stuff sold in packets.

3 cups water, soymilk, or other nondairy milk
1 cup old-fashioned rolled oats
Pinch salt

Put the water, oats, and salt in a medium saucepan and bring to a boil over medium-high heat. Decrease the heat to medium-low and cook, stirring occasionally, for about 10 minutes, until the oats are tender and creamy.

Tip: For added flavor and sweetness, stir ground cinnamon, raisins, or canned pineapple chunks into the oatmeal after it has finished cooking. Drizzle individual servings with maple syrup, agave nectar, or brown rice syrup.

Aunt Amanda's Pancakes

Makes 10 (3-inch) pancakes

ALTHOUGH THERE ARE some good packaged vegan pancake mixes available, it doesn't take long to make your own. Here's a simple recipe with no eggs or dairy.

1 cup whole wheat pastry flour
2 teaspoons aluminum-free baking powder
1 teaspoon evaporated cane juice
1/2 teaspoon ground cinnamon (optional)
1/4 teaspoon salt
1 cup soymilk
1 tablespoon plus 1 teaspoon canola oil
1 teaspoon vanilla extract (optional)

Put the flour, baking powder, evaporated cane juice, optional cinnamon, and salt in a large bowl and stir to mix thoroughly. Add the soymilk, 1 teaspoon of the oil, and the optional vanilla extract and whisk the ingredients until all the lumps are gone. Add water as needed to thin the batter to a pourable consistency.

Heat the remaining tablespoon of oil in a large skillet over medium-high heat. Test to see if the pan is hot enough by adding a drop of water. When the oil sizzles, decrease the heat to medium.

Using about 3 tablespoons of batter per pancake, add the batter to the skillet (2 or 3 pancakes will fit at a time) and cook until large bubbles begin to appear, about 2 minutes. Flip the pancakes and cook them on the second side for about 2 minutes, until golden brown. Repeat until all the batter is used.

Tofulicious Scramble

Makes 4 servings

THIS SCRAMBLE makes a great high-protein breakfast. Using fresh vegetables gives a contrast of textures, and you can vary the ingredients depending on what you have on hand.

1 tablespoon canola oil
1 onion, chopped
2 garlic cloves, minced
1 small zucchini, diced
1/2 large red or green bell pepper, diced
1/2 cup frozen peas
2 tablespoons reduced-sodium tamari
1/4 teaspoon ground turmeric
1 pound firm tofu, crumbled
1/4 teaspoon chili powder (optional)
Salt
Ground black pepper

Heat the oil in a medium skillet over medium heat. Add the onion and garlic and cook and stir for 5 to 10 minutes, until soft. Add the zucchini, pepper, and peas and cook for 3 to 5 minutes. Stir in the tamari.

Sprinkle the turmeric evenly over the tofu, then add to the vegetables and cook for 1 to 2 minutes to heat through. Add the optional chili powder and salt and pepper to taste. Stir thoroughly and serve immediately.

Tips:

➤ This scramble tastes great with veggie bacon or sausages for breakfast.

➤ For a hot lunch sandwich, spoon the tofu scramble into pita pockets that have been lined with lettuce leaves.

➤ Increase the chili powder to 1/2 teaspoon and serve the scramble with warmed black beans, salsa, and corn tortillas.

Red Potato Vampire Hash Browns

Makes 4 servings

RED POTATOES are perfect for hash browns because they hold their shape when cooked.

8 small red potatoes, sliced 1/4-inch thick
2 tablespoons canola oil
1 onion, chopped
Salt
Ground black pepper

Put the potatoes in a medium pot, add water to cover, bring to a boil, and cook for 5 minutes. Drain the pot and pat the potatoes dry with paper towels.

Heat the oil in a large skillet over medium heat. Add the onion and cook and stir for 5 to 10 minutes, until soft. Add the potatoes and cook for about 10 minutes, flipping the slices over occasionally, until they're browned on both sides. Sprinkle with salt and pepper to taste.

Tip: Boiling the potatoes briefly softens them so that they crisp more easily.

Pumpkin Patch Spice Muffins

Makes 10 muffins

THESE MOIST AND DELICIOUS fat-free muffins are great for breakfast or an afternoon snack.

2 cups whole wheat flour or whole wheat pastry flour
1/2 cup evaporated cane juice
1 tablespoon aluminum-free baking powder
1/2 teaspoon baking soda
1/2 teaspoon salt
1/2 teaspoon ground cinnamon
1/4 teaspoon ground nutmeg
1 (15-ounce) can solid-pack pumpkin
1/2 cup water
1/2 cup raisins

Preheat the oven to 375 degrees F. Spray 10 cups of a standard muffin tin with nonstick cooking spray and set aside.

Whisk the flour, evaporated cane juice, baking powder, baking soda, salt, cinnamon, and nutmeg together in a large bowl. Add the pumpkin, water, and raisins and stir just until incorporated.

Spoon the batter into the prepared muffin tin, filling to just below the tops. Bake for 25 to 30 minutes, until the tops of the muffins bounce back when pressed lightly. Remove from the oven and let stand for 5 minutes in the pan. Remove the muffins from the pan and cool on a rack. Store the cooled muffins in an airtight container.

Sides and Staples

Garlic Lover's Hummus

Makes 2 cups

THOUGH STORE-BOUGHT versions abound, making your own hummus is much less expensive and you can adjust the seasonings to suit your own taste.

1 (15-ounce) can chickpeas (garbanzo beans), drained, liquid reserved
¼ cup tahini
3 tablespoons lemon juice
1 large garlic clove, crushed
¼ teaspoon ground cumin
Chopped fresh parsley

Put the chickpeas, tahini, lemon juice, garlic, and cumin in a food processor or blender. Process until smooth, adding the reserved chickpea liquid as needed to adjust the consistency. Transfer the hummus into a serving bowl and garnish with parsley.

Tip: Leftover hummus will keep for 3 days stored in a covered container in the refrigerator.

Ali Baba's Ghanouj (eggplant dip)

Makes 1 cup

THE SECRET to the silky texture and smoky taste of this tasty dip is to cook the eggplant for a long time under high heat.

1 large eggplant (about 1 pound)
1 tablespoon olive oil
3 tablespoons lemon juice
2 tablespoons tahini
1 garlic clove, crushed
¾ teaspoon salt
1 tablespoon chopped fresh parsley (optional)

Preheat the broiler. Set an oven rack close to the broiler element, leaving enough room for the whole eggplant on a baking sheet.

Wash the eggplant and prick it all over with a fork. Brush the skin with the olive oil and place it on a baking sheet. Broil the eggplant for 30 to 45 minutes, turning every 10 minutes, until the skin is charred and the pulp is soft. Let it cool for 15 minutes.

Put the lemon juice, tahini, garlic, and salt in a blender and process for about 10 seconds. Cut the eggplant in half and scoop out the pulp. Add the eggplant to the blender and process until smooth.

Spoon the mixture into a serving bowl and sprinkle with the parsley, if using.

Tasty Tahini Sauce

Makes 1/2 cup

A STAPLE of Middle Eastern cooking, tahini is made from ground sesame seeds. Its slightly smoky flavor is perfectly complemented by the lemon and garlic in this sauce.

1/4 cup tahini
1 tablespoon lemon juice
1 tablespoon reduced-sodium tamari
1 tablespoon brown rice vinegar
1 garlic clove, minced
2 tablespoons water, or more as needed

Whisk the tahini, lemon juice, tamari, vinegar, garlic, and water together in a medium bowl until smooth. Whisk in additional water as needed to make the sauce pourable.

Tip: Serve with wedges of whole wheat pita bread or as a topping for falafel.

The Great American Coleslaw

Makes 6 servings

COLESLAW is a popular salad dish, and a great way to eat plenty of
nutritious cabbage.

1 cup vegan mayonnaise
3 tablespoons olive oil
2 tablespoons lemon juice
2 tablespoons tomato juice, or 1 tablespoon tomato purée (optional)
1 teaspoon dried basil (optional)
1 teaspoon dijon mustard (optional)
½ head green cabbage, finely sliced
1 large carrot, grated

To make the dressing, combine the mayonnaise, olive oil, and lemon juice in a
large bowl and stir until creamy. Add the optional ingredients as desired and stir
until well blended. Add the cabbage and carrot and stir to coat the vegetables
with the dressing. Cover and refrigerate for 1 hour before serving.

Basic Lentils

Makes 4 servings

SIMPLE, NOURISHING LENTILS are vegetarian comfort food. They taste great in
soups and stews, but they also have a wonderful flavor on their own.

1 cup dried brown or green lentils
2 cups water or vegetable broth
Salt

Put the lentils in a fine-mesh strainer and rinse under running water, then
transfer to a medium saucepan. Add the water and bring to a boil over medium-
high heat. Decrease the heat to medium-low, cover, and cook for about 20
minutes, until the lentils are tender. Season with salt to taste.

Mashed Potato Medley

Makes 6 servings

THIS VARIATION on the classic side dish adds a variety of root vegetables and cauliflower for added nutrition and flavor. When cooked, the vegetables take on a creamy texture.

1½ pounds yukon gold or white potatoes, chopped
8 ounces sweet potato, peeled and chopped
8 ounces parsnips, chopped
8 ounces cauliflower florets
1 cup soymilk (or other nondairy milk)
3 tablespoons nonhydrogenated vegan margarine
Salt
Ground black pepper

Bring a large pot of water to a boil. Add the potatoes and boil for 2 minutes. Add the parsnip and boil for 2 more minutes. Add the cauliflower, decrease the heat slightly, and cook for 6 to 10 minutes. Test the largest pieces of each vegetable by stabbing them with a sharp knife to see if they are soft. When all the vegetables are tender, drain the water and mash the vegetables together. Add the soymilk and margarine and mash until creamy. Season with salt and pepper to taste.

Tip: Serve with grilled vegetarian sausages, sliced mushrooms (cooked in a little water), and a steamed vegetable of your choice.

Roasted Vegetables

Makes as much as you like

ROASTING ROOT VEGETABLES gives them a luscious, crisp-chewy texture and caramelizes their natural sugars. This makes an excellent side dish for veggie burgers.

Potatoes, sweet potatoes, carrots, or parsnips, or a combination, scrubbed or peeled, cut in 1-inch pieces
Canola oil
Dried basil or thyme
Salt
Ground black pepper

Preheat the oven to 400 degrees F. Coat a baking sheet with oil or line it with parchment paper.

Bring a large pot of water to a boil. Add the potatoes and sweet potatoes and cook 5 minutes. Drain and pat dry. Put the potatoes in a large bowl, add the other vegetables, and drizzle with a little oil. Sprinkle with dried basil and season with salt and pepper to taste. Stir to coat all the vegetables with oil and seasonings, then turn out onto the prepared baking sheet and spread into a single layer. Bake for about 30 minutes, until tender and browned.

Tip: This recipe is easily adapted to make as many servings as you need. Figure on one to two vegetables per person.

Simple Brown Rice

Makes 4 servings

WITH ITS SATISFYING, slightly chewy texture, brown rice is the perfect accompaniment to a wide variety of great meals. Extra fiber and vitamins give it a nutritional edge over refined white rice.

1 cup brown rice
2 cups water
½ teaspoon salt

Put the rice in a fine-mesh strainer and rinse under running water, then transfer to a medium saucepan. Add the water and salt and bring to a boil over medium-high heat. Decrease the heat to low, cover, and cook for 35 to 45 minutes, until the rice is tender and the water is absorbed. Fluff with a fork before serving.

Quick Quinoa

Makes 4 servings

QUINOA IS A HIGH-PROTEIN GRAIN with a mildly nutty flavor and a delicate crunch. If you haven't tried it yet, you're in for a treat.

1 cup quinoa
1½ cups water or vegetable broth
Salt
Ground black pepper

Put the quinoa in a fine-mesh strainer and rinse thoroughly under running water, swishing the grains around with your fingers. Transfer to a medium saucepan, add the water, and bring to a boil over medium-high heat. Decrease the heat to medium-low, cover, and cook for 8 minutes, or until the grains look fluffy and little white threads curl around them. Drain any excess water. Season with salt and pepper to taste.

Say Cheeze Sauce

Makes 2 cups

THIS IS A SIMPLE cheese-style sauce, without the cheese. Nutritional yeast gives it a yellow hue and a cheeselike flavor. It can be poured over a variety of vegetables for a simple main course or thinned down with water and used as a gravy over meat-substitute dishes.

1/4 cup canola oil
1/4 cup whole wheat flour or whole wheat pastry flour
2 tablespoons nutritional yeast
2 cups soymilk
1 tablespoon reduced-sodium tamari
Salt

Put the oil in a medium saucepan over medium heat. Stir in the flour and nutritional yeast. Cook and stir for 1 to 2 minutes, until thick and doughy. Add more oil or flour if necessary to achieve a thick, doughy consistency. Gradually stir in the soymilk, mixing well to prevent lumps. Season with the tamari and salt to obtain a cheesy flavor.

Cauliflower Cheeze: Pour the sauce over steamed cauliflower, broccoli, and carrots and sprinkle a little nondairy cheese on top. Heat under a hot broiler until the sauce starts to bubble and the surface is lightly browned.

Mac 'n Cheeze: Pour the sauce over cooked pasta, such as macaroni, and heat under a hot broiler until the sauce starts to bubble.

Dinner

Kiss-the-Cook Mushroom Quiche

Makes 6 servings

TRY THIS RECIPE on someone you want to kiss!

1 tablespoon canola oil

4 ounces white or cremini mushrooms, sliced

1 (8–inch) pie crust, unbaked

1 pound silken tofu

2 tablespoons lemon juice

1 tablespoon reduced–sodium tamari

1 tablespoon dijon mustard

½ teaspoon garlic powder

2 ounces grated nondairy cheese

Preheat the oven to 375 degrees F.

Heat the oil in a medium skillet over medium-high heat. Add the sliced mushrooms and cook, stirring frequently, about 10 minutes or until browned. Transfer the mushrooms to the pie crust.

Put the tofu, lemon juice, tamari, mustard, and garlic powder in a food processor and process until creamy. Add the nondairy cheese and pulse two or three times to combine. Pour the mixture evenly over the mushrooms and bake for 50 to 55 minutes.

Tip: Almost any vegetable can be used in quiche. Substitute 1 chopped onion, 1 cup broccoli florets, or 1 cup corn kernels in place of the mushrooms.

"I'm Hungry" Hot Pot

Makes 4 servings

THIS IS A TASTY stick-to-the-ribs meal, suitable for the whole family.

1 cup cubed potatoes or sweet potatoes
1 cup sliced carrots
1 cup fusilli or other small pasta shape
1 cup frozen peas
1 tablespoon canola oil
1 cup chopped onion
2 cups Say Cheeze Sauce (page 143)
½ cup grated nondairy cheese

Preheat the broiler.

Bring two large pots of water to a boil. Put the potatoes and carrots in one pot and cook for 10 minutes. Put the pasta in the other pot and cook for 8 minutes. Add the peas to the pasta, bring back to a boil and cook for 2 more minutes. Drain the vegetables and pasta.

While the vegetables and pasta are cooking, put the oil in a skillet and cook the onion until soft and lightly browned. Transfer the onion to a 6-cup broiler-safe casserole dish. Stir in the potatoes, carrots, pasta, and peas. Pour the cheeze sauce over the vegetables and sprinkle the nondairy cheese on top. Broil until the sauce starts to bubble and the cheese turns light brown.

Tip: Serve with fresh steamed kale on the side.

Little Italy's Vegetable Lasagne

Makes 6 servings

THIS IS ANOTHER TASTY and nutritious dish to serve as a family meal. Serve with steamed fresh broccoli on the side.

9 lasagne noodles
1 tablespoon canola oil
1 onion, chopped
2 garlic cloves, minced
1 (14-ounce) container firm tofu, crumbled
1 (10-ounce) package frozen chopped spinach, thawed and squeezed dry
2 teaspoons dried basil
Salt
4 cups marinara sauce
½ cup grated nondairy cheese

Preheat the oven to 375 degrees F.

Fill a large pot with water and bring to a boil over high heat. Add the noodles and cook until just tender. Drain the noodles and rinse under cold running water.

While the noodles are cooking, heat the oil in a large skillet over medium heat. Add the onion and garlic and cook, stirring occasionally, for 5 to 7 minutes, or until the onion is translucent. Add the tofu, spinach, and basil and continue to cook, stirring occasionally, until the ingredients are heated through. Season with salt to taste.

Choose a deep baking dish (a 10 x 8 x 2-inch dish will work best). Coat the bottom with 1 cup of the marinara sauce. Arrange 3 noodles over the sauce in a single layer. Carefully spread half of the tofu mixture over the noodles. Spoon 1 more cup of the marinara sauce evenly over the tofu mixture. Add another layer of 3 more noodles. Carefully spread the remaining tofu mixture on top of them, and evenly cover with 1 more cup of the marinara sauce. Arrange the last 3 noodles on top, spread the remaining 1 cup of sauce evenly over the noodles, and sprinkle with the nondairy cheese. Bake for 30 minutes, or until the cheese has melted and is golden brown.

Tip: If you prefer a creamier lasagne, spread 1 cup of Say Cheeze Sauce (page 143) over each layer of the tofu mixture.

Beanie Rotini Pasta Marinara

Makes 4 servings

STORE-BOUGHT MARINARA sauce serves as the foundation for this nutritious meal, chock-full of vegetables and beans.

8 ounces rotini or other small pasta shape
1 tablespoon canola oil
½ onion, chopped
2 garlic cloves, minced
1 teaspoon dried basil
1 teaspoon dried thyme
2 small zucchini, chopped
1 small eggplant, peeled and chopped
1 (25-ounce) jar marinara sauce
1 (15-ounce) can black beans, drained and rinsed
4 large kale leaves, stemmed and chopped
Salt
Ground black pepper
1 tablespoon flaxseed oil

Bring a large pot of water to a boil. Add the rotini and cook for 10 minutes, or until just tender.

While the rotini is cooking, make the sauce. Heat the canola oil in a large skillet over medium heat. Add the onion, garlic, basil, and thyme and cook, stirring occasionally, for 5 to 7 minutes, until soft. Add the zucchini and eggplant and continue to cook, stirring, for about 8 minutes, or until the vegetables are tender. Add the marinara sauce, cover, and simmer for 10 minutes. Stir in the black beans and heat through. Stir in the kale and cook until wilted. Season with salt and pepper to taste.

Drain the rotini and toss with the flaxseed oil. Spoon the sauce over individual servings of rotini.

Tip: Flaxseed oil adds valuable omega-3 fatty acids to this meal, but if it's not available, toss the pasta with olive oil or canola oil.

Spaghetti with Besto Pesto Sauce

Makes 8 servings

PESTO MAKES A GREAT SAUCE for pasta. Unfortunately most commercial brands include cheese as a main ingredient. This sauce gets its creaminess from pine nuts or walnuts. It takes less than thirty minutes to prepare and is always a big hit.

1 pound spaghetti or linguini
1½ cups fresh basil leaves, loosely packed
¼ cup water
¼ cup pine nuts or chopped walnuts
1 tablespoon barley miso
1½ teaspoons olive oil
1 garlic clove, minced

Bring a large pot of water to a boil. Add the spaghetti and cook for 10 minutes, or until just tender.

While the spaghetti is cooking, make the pesto. Put the basil, water, 2 tablespoons of the nuts, the miso, oil, and garlic in a blender or food processor. Process until creamy. Add the remaining 2 tablespoons of nuts and process or pulse for a second or two, just until evenly incorporated.

Drain the spaghetti and return it to the pot. Add the pesto and toss until evenly distributed. Serve immediately.

Marco Polo Peanut Butter Pasta

Makes 4 servings

PEANUT SAUCE takes just minutes to prepare and gives spaghetti a whole new personality. Serve this spaghetti with lightly steamed vegetables.

8 ounces spaghetti
1/2 cup peanut butter
1 cup hot water
2 tablespoons reduced-sodium tamari
2 tablespoons seasoned rice vinegar
1 tablespoon evaporated cane juice
2 garlic cloves, minced
1/2 teaspoon ground ginger

Bring a large pot of water to a boil. Add the spaghetti and cook for 10 minutes, or until just tender.

While the pasta is cooking, make the sauce. Put the peanut butter, water, tamari, vinegar, evaporated cane juice, garlic, and ginger in a large saucepan and whisk to blend. Cook the sauce over low heat for about 5 minutes, or until slightly thickened. Drain the spaghetti, add it to the sauce, toss to blend.

Secret Swiss Chard Sauté

Makes 4 servings

THIS RECIPE USES FRESH tomatoes instead of marinara sauce, which gives it a lighter flavor and texture.

8 ounces penne or other tube-shaped pasta
1 tablespoon canola oil
1 onion, chopped
2 garlic cloves, minced
1 pound roma tomatoes, chopped
1 bunch swiss chard, washed, stemmed, and sliced into 1-inch-wide strips
Ground black pepper
Grated nondairy parmesan cheese

Bring a large pot of water to a boil and cook the penne for 10 minutes, or until just tender.

While the pasta is cooking, heat the oil in a large skillet over medium heat. Add the onion and garlic and cook, stirring occasionally, for 5 to 7 minutes, until soft. Add the tomatoes and heat through, then add the chard.

Drain the penne and toss with a little flaxseed oil (or other oil) to prevent sticking. Spoon the cooked chard mixture over individual portions of penne and top with black pepper and cheese to taste.

Tips:

➤ For a protein boost, add one (15-ounce) can of cannellini beans, drained and rinsed.
➤ If fresh tomatoes are not available, substitute one (14.5-ounce) can of diced tomatoes with their juice.
➤ It may seem as if you have too much chard when you first add it to the skillet, but like spinach, chard collapses into a much smaller volume when cooked.

Veggie Sloppy Joes

Makes 4 servings

WHEN YOU HAVE FAMILY members asking for meat, this dish will fool them into thinking it's spaghetti sauce with ground turkey. Although tempeh may look like turkey, it doesn't have any saturated fat or cholesterol, and it's much more nutritious.

1 cup water

3 tablespoons reduced-sodium tamari

1 (8-ounce) package tempeh, crumbled

1 tablespoon canola oil

1 onion, chopped

1 garlic clove, minced

8 ounces cremini mushrooms, sliced (optional)

2 large carrots, chopped (optional)

1 (25-ounce) jar marinara sauce

1 cup frozen peas (optional)

4 whole wheat hamburger buns

Combine the water and tamari in a medium bowl. Add the tempeh and let it marinate for 30 minutes, if time permits.

Heat the oil in a large skillet over medium heat. Add the onion and garlic and cook and stir for 5 to 10 minutes, until the onion is soft and lightly browned. Add the optional mushrooms and carrots and cook for about 5 minutes, stirring occasionally. Drain the tempeh and add it to the skillet. Cook for 5 to 10 minutes, stirring frequently, until brown. Add the marinara sauce and bring to a boil over medium-high heat. Decrease the heat to medium, cover, and simmer for about 7 minutes. Add the optional peas and cook for 3 minutes longer. Serve on the hamburger buns.

Tips:

➤ The optional vegetables in this recipe add extra nutrition. You can substitute equal amounts of other vegetables, such as zucchini or bell peppers, for the ones listed here.

➤ To save time, prepare the vegetables and start cooking them while the tempeh is marinating.

South-of-the-Border Vegetarian Chili

Makes 4 servings

THERE ARE MANY BRANDS of canned vegetarian chili available. Here's a simple recipe to make for yourself. Note that black beans and red beans are a lot more digestible than the classic kidney beans. TVP (textured vegetable protein) would also work well if you don't have tempeh available.

1 tablespoon canola oil
1 small onion, chopped
1 garlic clove, minced
1 tablespoon reduced-sodium tamari
1½ teaspoons chili powder
1½ teaspoons evaporated cane juice
1 (8-ounce) package tempeh, crumbled
1 (14.5-ounce) can diced tomatoes, undrained
½ cup tomato purée
1 (15-ounce) can red beans, drained and rinsed
1 (15-ounce) can black beans, drained and rinsed
Salt

Heat the oil in a large skillet. Add the onion and garlic and cook and stir for 5 to 10 minutes, until soft. Stir in the tamari, chili powder, and evaporated cane juice and mix well. Add the crumbled tempeh and mix well to coat the tempeh. Add the diced tomatoes and tomato purée and stir until well blended. Add the red beans and black beans. Cover and simmer for 30 minutes. Add salt and additional evaporated cane juice or chili powder to taste.

Tip: Serve in a large wrap or corn tortillas, with cooked rice and salad, or with a baked potato.

Savory Indian Curry Base

Makes 4 servings

THIS AROMATIC MIXTURE of onion, garlic, and warm spices forms the base for Benny Bengali's Indian Curry (page 156), The Yogi's Favorite Braised Vegetable Curry (page 157), and Chandra's Chickpea Curry (page 158).

1 tablespoon canola oil
1 onion, chopped
2 garlic cloves, minced
1 tablespoon peeled and grated fresh ginger (optional)
2 teaspoons ground coriander
2 teaspoons ground cumin
1 teaspoon chili powder
1/2 teaspoon ground turmeric
Salt
Ground black pepper

Heat the oil in a large skillet over medium heat. Add the onion and garlic and cook, stirring occasionally, for 5 to 7 minutes, until soft. Add the optional ginger, coriander, cumin, chili powder, turmeric, and salt and pepper to taste and mix well. Cook, stirring frequently, for 3 to 5 minutes.

Lucky Lee's Tofu and Vegetable Stir-Fry

Makes 4 servings

A STIR-FRY is a quick and easy way to cook a lot of vegetables.

1½ cups brown rice
3 cups water
1 teaspoon salt
1 (14-ounce) container firm tofu
2 tablespoons canola oil
Reduced-sodium tamari
1 onion, chopped
1 garlic clove, minced
1 large carrot, sliced
1 zucchini, quartered lengthwise and sliced
1 red bell pepper, chopped
4 ounces sugar snap peas, tips removed

Put the rice in a fine-mesh strainer and rinse under running water. Transfer to a medium saucepan. Add the water and salt and bring to a boil over medium-high heat. Decrease the heat to low, cover, and cook for 35 to 45 minutes, until the rice is tender and the water is absorbed.

Slice the tofu crosswise into 6 thick slices. Wrap the slices in paper towels and press to soak up the excess water. Remove the paper towels, stack the slices, then cut the tofu into cubes. Heat 1 tablespoon of the oil in a large skillet over medium heat. Add the tofu and sprinkle with tamari to taste, then turn the cubes over and sprinkle again with tamari to taste. Cook for 8 to 10 minutes, turning the cubes until they are browned on all sides.

Heat the remaining tablespoon of oil in a skillet over medium heat. Add the onion and garlic and cook and stir for 5 to 10 minutes, until soft. Add the carrot, zucchini, bell pepper, and sugar snap peas and cook and stir until just tender. Sprinkle tamari over the vegetables to taste.

Divide the rice among individual plates, add a large spoonful of the vegetables, then top with the tofu.

Tip: To make preparation easier, replace the fresh vegetables with a 1-pound package of frozen mixed vegetables.

Quick Red Lentils (*dal*)

Makes 4 servings

LENTILS ARE EXCEEDINGLY nutritious, very tasty, and easily digested by almost everyone. There are many different kinds of lentils, each having a slightly different flavor. Red lentils collapse when cooked to form a smooth paste, which can be served alone, added to a basic curry, or blended into a vegetable curry.

1 cup dried red lentils
2 cups vegetable broth
Salt

Put the lentils in a fine-mesh strainer and rinse under running water. Transfer to a medium saucepan. Add the water and bring to a boil over medium-high heat. Decrease the heat to medium-low, cover, and cook for about 20 minutes, until the lentils are tender. Season with salt to taste.

Tips:

➤ You can use premade vegetable broth, one or two vegetable broth cubes, or tablespoons of powder dissolved in 2 cups of boiling water, or leftover vegetable cooking water.

➤ Serve these lentils over rice, with steamed vegetables on the side, for a very simple meal.

Benny Bengali's Indian Curry

Makes 4 servings

THE SIMPLE ADDITION of diced tomatoes gives this easy curry a real flavor boost.

1 tablespoon canola oil
1 recipe Savory Indian Curry Base (page 153)
1 (14.5-ounce) can diced tomatoes, undrained
1 recipe Quick Red Lentils (page 155)

Heat the oil in a large skillet over medium heat. Stir in the curry base and tomatoes with their juice. Decrease the heat to medium-low, cover, and cook for 10 minutes. Stir the lentils into the curry mixture and cook to heat through.

Tips:

➢ If you prepare the curry base just before you make this recipe, keep the curry base in the skillet so you don't need to dirty another pan.

➢ If time permits, prepare the curry base in advance (even several days ahead) and refrigerate it until you are ready to make this recipe.

➢ Serve this curry over brown rice.

The Yogi's Favorite Braised Vegetable Curry

Makes 4 servings

THIS WARM AND LIGHTLY spiced curry offers a variety of vegetables to provide a good balance of nutrition.

1 tablespoon canola oil
1 recipe Savory Indian Curry Base (page 153)
1 sweet potato, yam, or parsnip, peeled and chopped
1 zucchini or yellow squash, chopped
2 cups vegetable broth
1 cup Quick Red Lentils (page 155)
Leafy greens (such as kale, collards, chard, or spinach), stemmed and chopped

Heat the oil in a large skillet over medium heat and add the curry base. Add the sweet potato and zucchini and stir to coat the vegetables. Add the broth and bring to a boil over medium-high heat. Decrease the heat to medium-low, cover, and simmer for 10 minutes, until the sweet potato is cooked. Stir the lentils into the mixture, then stir in the greens and cook for 2 to 12 minutes, until the greens are tender.

Tips:

➤ If you prepare the curry base just before you make this recipe, keep the curry base in the skillet so you don't need to dirty another pan.

➤ If time permits, prepare the curry base in advance (even several days ahead) and refrigerate it until you are ready to make this recipe.

➤ Instead of mixing the lentils in with the vegetables, keep the lentils on the side and serve them as two separate dishes.

➤ This curry tastes great served over brown rice.

Chandra's Chickpea Curry

Makes 4 servings

CAULIFLOWER, LIKE BROCCOLI, is a cruciferous vegetable that contains powerful health-protecting nutrients. Its mild flavor makes it the perfect vegetable to soak up the savory sauce in this curry.

1 recipe Savory Indian Curry Base (page 153)
1 (14.5-ounce) can diced tomatoes, undrained, or tomato sauce
½ head cauliflower, separated into small florets
1 large carrot, sliced
4 ounces cremini mushrooms, quartered
1 (15-ounce) can chickpeas, drained and rinsed

Put the curry base in a large skillet. Add the tomatoes with their juice and the cauliflower and cook for 5 minutes. Add the carrot, mushrooms, and enough water, if needed, to cover the vegetables. Stir to mix well and cook for 10 minutes. Stir in the chickpeas and simmer for 5 to 10 minutes, until the vegetables are tender and the chickpeas are heated through.

Tips:

➤ If you prepare the curry base just before you make this recipe, keep the curry base in the skillet so you don't need to dirty another pan.

➤ If time permits, prepare the curry base in advance (even several days ahead) and refrigerate it until you are ready to make this recipe.

➤ To save time, use one 15-ounce jar of Indian nondairy curry sauce in this recipe instead of the curry base.

➤ Serve this curry over brown rice, with a steamed green vegetable, such as kale, on the side.

Taste of Thailand Tofu Curry

Makes 4 servings

COCONUT MILK makes this curry creamy and rich and balances the spicy heat of
the curry paste.

1 tablespoon canola oil
1 tablespoon red, yellow, or green Thai curry paste
1 (15-ounce) can lite coconut milk
1 tablespoon reduced-sodium tamari
1 tablespoon evaporated cane juice or other sweetener, plus more
as needed
Lime juice (optional)
1 (14-ounce) container firm tofu, blotted dry and cut in cubes

Heat the oil in a large skillet over medium heat. Blend in the curry paste until it
emits a fragrant aroma. Stir the coconut milk into the paste until well blended.
Add the tamari and evaporated cane juice and stir to mix. Taste the sauce and
add the optional lime juice and additional evaporated cane juice to taste. Add
the tofu and bring to a boil. Decrease the heat to medium-low and cook for 5
minutes, stirring occasionally, until the tofu is heated through.

Tips:

➤ For a quicker curry, substitute one 12-ounce jar of Thai curry simmer sauce
   for the coconut milk and curry paste.
➤ Serve the tofu curry over brown rice and steamed vegetables.

Vinnie's Vegetable Risotto

Makes 6 servings

THIS CLASSIC ITALIAN DISH is made with arborio rice, a short-grain rice with a high starch content, which gives risotto a creamy consistency.

4 cups vegetable broth
1 cup arborio rice
1 onion, finely chopped
2 cups broccoli florets
1 cup finely chopped zucchini
1 cup frozen corn, thawed
1 cup finely chopped red bell pepper
1 cup finely chopped green bell pepper
2 cups chopped fresh spinach
1 tablespoon reduced-sodium tamari
Ground black pepper

Put 3½ cups of the broth in a large saucepan and bring to a boil. Stir in the rice, decrease the heat to low, and cook, stirring frequently, until the broth is absorbed, about 15 minutes.

While the rice is cooking, heat the remaining ½ cup of broth in a large nonstick skillet over medium heat. Add the onion, broccoli, zucchini, corn, and red and green bell peppers and cook, stirring occasionally, for 10 minutes. Stir in the spinach and tamari and cook for about 3 minutes, or until the spinach is wilted. Add the vegetable mixture to the rice and stir to combine. Season with black pepper to taste.

Tip: Substitute an equal amount of pearl barley for the arborio rice for a less creamy but equally delicious risotto.

Desserts

Creamy Chocolate Dream Pudding

Makes 4 (½-cup) servings

SILKEN TOFU makes it easy to prepare a smooth and creamy chocolate pudding without using cream.

1 pound soft silken tofu
⅓ to ½ cup maple syrup
2 tablespoons cocoa powder
1 teaspoon vanilla extract
¼ teaspoon salt

Put all the ingredients in a blender and process until completely smooth. Spoon the mixture into four small bowls. Chill well before serving.

Tip: For a richer pudding, process ½ cup chocolate chips, melted, with the other ingredients.

Grandma's Apple Crisp

Makes 10 (3/4-cup) servings

THIS CLASSIC DESSERT is quick to throw together and so good for you that you could eat it for breakfast.

4 large tart apples, peeled, cored, and thinly sliced
3/4 cup evaporated cane juice or other sweetener
1/2 cup whole wheat pastry flour
1 teaspoon ground cinnamon
1 1/2 cups old-fashioned rolled oats
1/3 cup nonhydrogenated vegan margarine

Preheat the oven to 350 degrees F.

Toss the apples with 1/2 cup of the evaporated cane juice, 1 tablespoon of the flour, and the cinnamon. Spread the apples evenly in a 9 x 13-inch baking dish.

Mix the oats with the remaining 1/4 cup of evaporated cane juice and 7 tablespoons of flour. Add the margarine and use your fingers or a fork to blend the ingredients together until the mixture is uniformly crumbly. Sprinkle the oat mixture evenly over the apples. Bake for 45 minutes, or until lightly browned. Let the apple crisp stand for 10 minutes before serving.

Tips:
➤ For extra nutrients, leave the peels on the apples.
➤ If you like, serve the crisp warm with nondairy vanilla ice cream.

Passion for Pumpkin Pie

Makes 8 servings

THIS IS THE EASIEST and most healthful pumpkin pie recipe ever.

18 to 20 ounces lite silken tofu
1 (15-ounce) can solid-pack pumpkin
2/3 cup brown rice syrup or other thick liquid sweetener
1 tablespoon pumpkin pie spice
1 teaspoon vanilla extract
1 (9-inch) deep-dish pie crust, unbaked

Preheat the oven to 350 degrees F.

Put the tofu in a food processor or blender and process until smooth. Add the pumpkin, syrup, pumpkin pie spice, and vanilla extract and process until the ingredients are completely incorporated, scraping down the bowl if necessary. Pour into the pie crust and bake for about 1 hour, until the filling is fairly firm but jiggles slightly when shaken. (The filling will continue to firm up as it cools.) Cool completely before serving.

Tip: A mixture of 1½ teaspoons ground cinnamon, 3/4 teaspoon ground ginger, and 1/4 teaspoon ground cloves may be substituted for the pumpkin pie spice.

Chocolate Bonbons

Makes about 40 bonbons

WHEN YOU'VE GOT to have chocolate, these bonbons will just melt in your mouth.

1/4 cup brown rice syrup
1/4 cup natural almond or peanut butter
1 1/2 tablespoons unsweetened cocoa or carob powder
1 tablespoon organic canola or safflower oil
1/2 teaspoon vanilla extract
2 brown rice cakes, finely crushed, or 1 1/4 cups puffed or crisped brown rice cereal

Line a baking sheet with waxed paper or parchment paper.

Put the syrup, almond butter, cocoa, and oil in a medium saucepan and warm over low heat, stirring until completely combined. Remove from the heat and stir in the vanilla extract. Using a sturdy wooden spoon, stir in the crushed rice cakes until thoroughly incorporated. Let the mixture cool until it can be handled easily. Working with 1 tablespoon of the mixture at a time, roll it between your hands into 1-inch balls. As you work, place each ball on the prepared baking sheet. Transfer to an airtight container and store at room temperature.

Wild Oatmeal Chocolate Chip Cookies

Makes about 12 (3-inch) cookies

THESE TASTY COOKIES are quick and easy to make.

1½ cups old-fashioned rolled oats
½ cup whole wheat pastry flour
¼ teaspoon salt
⅓ cup canola oil
¼ cup brown rice syrup
1 teaspoon vanilla extract
⅓ cup chopped walnuts
⅓ cup chocolate or carob chips

Preheat the oven to 350 degrees F. Oil a baking sheet or line it with parchment paper and set aside.

Put the oats, flour, and salt in a medium bowl and mix well. Combine the oil, syrup, and vanilla extract in a small bowl and stir until well blended. Gradually stir the wet ingredients into the dry ingredients until completely incorporated. Stir in the walnuts and chocolate chips. Using wet hands and working with about 2 rounded tablespoons of dough at a time, form the dough into balls and place on the prepared baking sheet. Flatten the dough balls until they are about 3 inches across. Bake for 15 to 20 minutes, until crisp and golden around the edges. Cool on a wire rack.

Resources

Websites

If you google a particular topic, you may be overwhelmed by the choice of websites available to you. People often have their own agendas or opinions, which they promote on websites. These may or may not be based on facts, so you can find websites that say all kinds of things, including the exact opposite of what's stated in this book. There won't be any reliable facts to back up their statements, but they'll look very convincing. Don't be fooled. If you want to know more about a specific topic, here are some websites we trust that are worth reading:

Health
Physicians Committee for Responsible Medicine
www.pcrm.org
The Physicians Committee for Responsible Medicine provides a wealth of reliable nutritional information on the many advantages of a vegetarian diet, communicated in everyday language.

John McDougall
www.drmcdougall.com
John McDougall, MD, is a well-known expert in nutrition and leader in the field of vegetarian nutrition research. There's lots of information here in an easy-to-understand form.

Animals
The Humane Society
www.humanesociety.org
The Humane Society of the United States is the largest and most broadly supported animal welfare organization in the country. Look for information on animal issues, such as factory farming, on their issue page, and practical information on becoming a vegetarian on their eating page.

Jane Goodall

www.janegoodall.org

Jane Goodall is a world-famous anthropologist and vegetarian. Look under Harvest for Hope for information about how a vegetarian diet helps your health, the animals, and the environment. Young people will be especially interested in the Roots and Shoots Foundation.

Environment
The Worldwatch Institute

www.worldwatch.org

The Worldwatch Institute is a very highly respected environmental organization. It advocates sustainability through moving toward a vegetarian diet. This organization has highlighted livestock agriculture as the prime cause of global warming.

World Religions
Christian Vegetarian Association

www.all-creatures.org/cva/default.htm

The Christian Vegetarian Association is a nondenominational organization promoting a vegetarian diet from a position of faith.

Indian Vegetarians

www.youngindianvegetarians.co.uk

The followers of the different religions of India will find a wealth of information and support here, along with a free newsletter.

Islam Vegetarians

www.islamveg.com

Young Muslims will find this a valuable site for promoting a vegetarian diet based on the Koran and *hadith*.

Jewish Vegetarians

www.jewishveg.com

The Jewish Vegetarians of North America sponsor this site, which provides information, a newsletter, and support for Jewish vegetarians. Young vegetarians will be especially interested in the video "A Sacred Duty" available on the site.

Recipe Websites

The Vegetarian Times

www.vegetariantimes.com

Vegetarian Times magazine maintains a huge database of both vegetarian and vegan recipes, plus weekly e-newsletters. Get a free subscription to their high-quality magazine when you join Vegetarians of Washington at www.vegofwa. org.

NutritionMD

www.nutritionmd.org

The Physicians Committee for Responsible Medicine operates NutritionMD, which offers help and support to people who want to go vegetarian by providing meal plans, advice, and a huge supply of vegan recipes.

E-newsletters

The Vegetarian Page

To sign up visit www.vegofwa.org/newsflashsignup.html

The Vegetarian Page is a free newsletter produced by Vegetarians of Washington, covering the latest news and many benefits of a vegetarian diet, plus information about ingredients and tasty recipes.

The VegE-News

www.vege-news.com

A Canadian newsletter, The VegE-News covers the latest information on a wide range of vegetarian topics from an international perspective.

Books

There are hundreds of books on vegetarian topics. Here are the ones we can particularly recommend.

General Vegetarian Books

The Vegetarian Solution

Stewart Rose (Healthy Living Publications, 2007)

Written by the vice president of Vegetarians of Washington, *The Vegetarian Solution* answers the questions most frequently asked by its members and the general public. A comprehensive look at the many benefits of a vegetarian diet written in a light-hearted and supportive style, this book provides up-to-date information on how a vegetarian diet can improve your health and the world you live in. It has been enthusiastically endorsed by several medical doctors and makes scientific topics accessible in an easy-to-understand way.

101 Reasons Why I'm a Vegetarian
Pamela Rice (Lantern Books, 2004)
If you're looking for more reasons to give up meat, *101 Reasons Why I'm a Vegetarian* is an enlightening book to dip into. The "reasons" focus on environmental and animal cruelty issues, although health, nutrition, social, and economic concerns are also addressed. It is based on a popular brochure that Pamela Rice distributed in New York for many years.

The New Becoming Vegetarian: The Essential Guide to a Healthy Vegetarian Diet
Vesanto Melina, MS, RD, Brenda Davis, RD (Book Publishing Company, 2003)
The New Becoming Vegetarian provides a detailed look at all the nutritional requirements of a vegetarian diet, with lots of valuable information about the health-supporting benefits of a vegetarian diet added in. It also contains useful hints on handling various social situations vegetarian-style, along with meal planning ideas and lots of recipes.

Becoming Vegan: The Complete Guide to Adopting a Healthy Plant-Based Diet
Brenda Davis, RD, Vesanto Melina, MS, RD (Book Publishing Company, 2000)
Becoming Vegan is similar to *Becoming Vegetarian*, but puts more emphasis on how to avoid dairy products, where to get vitamin B_{12}, and how to create balanced vegan diets for infants, children, and seniors. Other useful topics include considerations for pregnancy and breast-feeding, coping with weight issues and eating disorders, and achieving peak performance as a vegan athlete.

Vegan in 30 Days: Get Healthy. Save the World
Sarah Taylor (Taylor Presentations, Inc., 2008)
Vegan in 30 Days will help you reach your goal of becoming vegan in healthful and fun ways. Included are over a dozen starter recipes for flavorful, easy-to-make dishes. Weekly assignments keep you actively involved in the process, and lists of resources help keep you motivated. Guidelines for social engagements, like hosting or attending a dinner party or eating at a restaurant, show you how to make others aware of your diet without offending them and their dietary preferences.

Specific Issue Books

Dr. Dean Ornish's Program for Reversing Heart Disease: The Only System Scientifically Proven to Reverse Heart Disease Without Drugs or Surgery
Dean Ornish, MD (Ivy Books, 1996)
Young people take note: your arteries begin to clog in childhood. *Dr. Dean Ornish's Program for Reversing Heart Disease* tackles the biggest health issue of all: heart disease. Texas cardiologist Dean Ornish was the first to prove that not only would a vegetarian diet prevent the formation of clogged arteries that leads to heart attacks, but that a vegetarian diet could actually clear out arteries that were already clogged. Ornish is an internationally recognized leader in the field of vegetarian nutrition.

Dr. Neal Barnard's Program for Reversing Diabetes: The Scientifically Proven System for Reversing Diabetes without Drugs
Neal D. Barnard, MD (Rodale Books, 2007)
The incidence of diabetes is rising rapidly especially among young people. *Dr. Neal Barnard's Program for Reversing Diabetes* tells readers how they can avoid diabetes through nutrition, and even reverse diabetes by following a vegan diet. Barnard is the president of the Physicians Committee for Responsible Medicine.

Diet for Transcendence: Vegetarianism and the World Religions
Steven Rosen (Torchlight Publishing; revised edition, 1997)
In *Diet for Transcendence*, a well-researched and reliable book, the author shows the rich history of vegetarianism among different world religions. Written in bite-sized chapters, this book will surprise anyone who thinks that Western religion hasn't supported the vegetarian diet.

Happier Meals: Rethinking the Global Meat Industry
Danielle Nierenberg (Worldwatch Institute, 2005)
Happier Meals is a gem. Few books cover the global perspective as well as this one. Here you will discover how a vegetarian diet is the solution to global public health and environmental problems.

Harvest for Hope: A Guide to Mindful Eating
Jane Goodall (Warner Books, 2005)
Written by a famous and well-respected anthropologist, Jane Goodall, *Harvest for Hope* explains how a vegetarian diet is both the most natural and the most health-promoting diet to follow. Additional material on ethics in agriculture and organics makes this a valuable and reliable resource.

Cookbooks

Kids Can Cook: Vegetarian Recipes
Dorothy R. Bates (Book Publishing Company, Revised Edition, 2001)
Designed for teenagers, *Kids Can Cook* is full of fun and easy vegetarian recipes to get you started. These recipes were all developed in cooking classes for teens, so they've been tested on kids by kids. There are hints and tips throughout for the beginning cook.

Student's Go Vegan Cookbook: Over 135 Quick, Easy, Cheap, and Tasty Vegan Recipes
Carole Raymond, (Three Rivers Press, 2006)
With lots of helpful tips for stocking your kitchen and planning your meals, the *Student's Go Vegan Cookbook* is a valuable source of information. The recipes are straightforward, without expensive ingredients but with plenty of variety.

The Veg-Feasting Cookbook: Favorite Recipes From Local Restaurants and Leading Chefs in the Pacific Northwest
Vegetarians of Washington (Book Publishing Company, 2005)
The Veg-Feasting Cookbook includes all the recipes you'll ever need. If you want to impress your friends by trying out different cuisines, such as African, Indian, or Thai food, you'll find just what you're looking for. The recipes were provided by the best vegetarian and veg-friendly restaurants throughout Washington State and Oregon, plus some of the region's leading cookbook authors, who gave cooking demonstrations at Vegfest, a health-promoting vegetarian food festival held in Seattle each spring.

Local Bounty: Seasonal Vegan Recipes
Devra Gartenstein (Book Publishing Company, 2008)
If you'd like to try eating with the seasons, choosing your recipes to use the produce available at a given time of year in order to minimize the travel costs of your produce, you'll find *Local Bounty* invaluable.

I Can't Believe It's Tofu!
Marilyn Joyce, PhD, RD
I Can't Believe It's Tofu! takes the "Yuk!" out of tofu. It's for anyone who can't get past the look and taste of tofu, or who doesn't know how to use it, but wants to have its healthful benefits. This is the most complete and easy-to-use tofu guide available. It answers every question you have about what tofu is, how it is made, its numerous health benefits, and how to incorporate it daily into your diet as part of a delicious, nutritious eating plan. What sets this book apart from all the rest is its absolute simplicity of use—no recipe takes more than five minutes to prepare. Available from www.marilynjoyce.com/book.html

Tofu, Quick and Easy
Louise Hagler (Book Publishing Company, Revised Edition, 2001)
Tofu is an extremely versatile form of protein for vegetarians. If you'd like to include more tofu in your diet, *Tofu, Quick and Easy* has plenty of quick, easy recipes, including everything from mock chicken salad and enchiladas to almond cheesecake.

Vegan Bites: Recipes for Singles
Beverly Lynn Bennett (Book Publishing Company, 2008)
Focusing on quick, easy vegan meals for just one person, *Vegan Bites* is really helpful when you want to keep the prep time and the leftovers to a minimum. There are more than one hundred easy-to-make recipes, encompassing a wide variety of foods and cuisines, with selections for every skill level and schedule.

Vegetarians of Washington

Vegetarians of Washington is one of the largest vegetarian societies in the United States. We hold monthly dinners and free classes, give talks to interested groups, and give out information about the benefits of vegetarian food at various public events. Our books are written to help people learn about the benefits of vegetarian food, discover new recipes to cook, and find restaurants where they can enjoy delicious vegetarian meals. Our main event of the year is Vegfest, the largest vegetarian food festival in the United States.

Our monthly dinners in Seattle are catered by a different restaurant or chef each month, so you can try a variety of vegetarian cuisines, such as Indian one month, Mexican the next. These dinners are warm, friendly events where people of all ages and walks of life can meet and enjoy a meal together. There's always a short but informative speech about an interesting vegetarian topic, and lots of delicious food.

Our free classes typically include an informative nutrition class, which takes you by the hand and guides you through the many nutritional and other benefits of a vegetarian diet, based on our acclaimed book *The Vegetarian Solution*. Following this, a cooking class provides hints and tips on preparing some key vegetarian ingredients, and lots of delicious samples to taste. In one afternoon you can learn all you need to know about how and why to go vegetarian, and get all your questions answered.

This is the fifth book we have published. Our first book, *Veg-Feasting in the Pacific Northwest*, was a guidebook to vegetarian and veg-friendly restaurants and natural food stores throughout Washington and Oregon, helping people to find a good place to eat or to buy food when they're out and about. This book was updated and republished a few years later as *Vegetarian Pacific Northwest*. We invited the restaurants in these guidebooks to share their best recipes with us, enabling us to compile a wonderful cookbook, *The Veg-Feasting Cookbook*, full of interesting and delicious recipes from many different cuisines.

The Vegetarian Solution, by Stewart Rose, provides a comprehensive look at all the many reasons to go vegetarian. With a particular emphasis on the health benefits, backed up by many detailed reference studies, this book provides an up-to-date look at how you can improve your health and the world you live in. We have also compiled a series of informative brochures, which we provide free of charge at events, and which can be downloaded and printed from our website.

Vegfest, a health-promoting vegetarian food festival held at the Seattle Center in the spring of each year, brings together the whole vegetarian community to showcase the many types of vegetarian food available. Doctors give informative talks on nutrition, chefs and cookbook authors demonstrate how to cook vegetarian food, and clowns perform for the kids, but best of all, there are more than 700 different kinds of foods to try.

Vegetarians of Washington is a warm and friendly organization where we encourage people to proceed at their own pace and do the best they can while making positive changes to their diets. You don't have to be a vegetarian to come to any of our events or even to join our organization. To learn more, or to join, visit our website: www.VegofWA.org.

Index

C

cabbage, 85, 116,
    coleslaw recipe, 139
calcium, 30, 83-85, 122
calories, 25, 28, 56-57
cancer, 29, 36-38
carnivore, 23-24
carrots, 126,
    recipes, 141, 145, 151
casein, 88, 122
cashew *(see also nuts)*
    butter, 122
    protein in, 80
Catholic, Roman, 61
cauliflower, 125,
    recipes, 140, 143, 158
cereal, 105, 114
chard, Swiss, 116, 126,
    recipe, 150
cheese,
    alternatives, 117, 122
    cholesterol in, 33
cheeze sauce recipe, 143
chemicals, toxic, 29, 36
chicken
    cholesterol in, 30
    eating, 82
    raising, 43-44
    saturated fat in, 34

chickpeas, *(see also beans)*
    in hummus, 121
    protein in, 80
    recipes, 136, 158
childhood diabetes, 31
chili,
    canned, 107, 111
    recipe, 152
Chinese restaurants, 102
chocolate, 78, 109, 110
    recipes, 161, 164, 165
cholesterol, 22-23, 32-35, 38
Christians, 62
cigarettes, 15-16, 35, 38
cinnamon, *(see spices)*
cocoa powder, 110
coconut *(see also nuts)*
    milk, 111
    yogurt, 79, 107
coleslaw recipe, 139
collard greens, 85, 116, 126
concentration, 26
Confucius, 62, 65
cookbooks, recommended, 172
cookies, 108, 109
    chocolate chip recipe, 165
coriander *(see spices)*

P

vegetable, *(see also individual vegetables)*

    calcium in, 85

    in diet, 124

    oil, 127

    preparation of, 125

    protein in, 80

    roasted, 141

    types of, 78, 116

vegetarian movement, 75

Vegetarians of Washington, 175-176

Vegetarian Times, the, 169

Vietnamese restaurants, 103

vinegar, 112

vitamins, 29, 89

W

waffles, 106

walnuts, *(see also nuts)*

    omega-3 oils in, 83, 113

    recipes, 148, 165

water,

    to drink, 78, 84, 86, 111

    pollution, 49, 53

    resources, 51-52

websites, 17, 167

weight, 23, 25

Weismuller, Johnny, 27

Wesley, John, 12, 61

wheat, *(see also grains, whole)*

    allergies, 88

    germ, 113

    gluten, 117, 120

    growing, 56, 58

    protein in, 80-81

    whole flour, 110, 123

White, Ellen G, 12, 61

Wiig, Kristen, 13

Williams, Ricky, 13

Worldwatch Institute, the, 168, 171

Y

yams, *(see vegetables)*

yogurt, 107, 117

Z

zucchini, 124-126

    recipes,

        pasta marinara, 147,

        tofu scramble, 133,

        vegetable curry, 157

        vegetable risotto, 160

        vegetable stir-fry, 154,

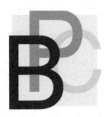

BOOK PUBLISHING COMPANY

since 1974—books that educate, inspire, and empower

To find your favorite vegetarian and soyfood products online, visit:
www.healthy-eating.com

Also by the Vegetarians of Washington

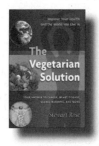

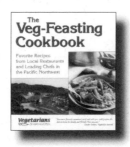

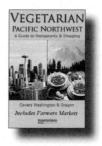

The Vegetarian Solution
978-1-57067-205-7 $12.95

The Veg-Feasting Cookbook
978-1-57067-178-4 $18.95

Vegetarian Pacific Northwest
978-1-57067-211-8 $14.95

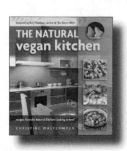

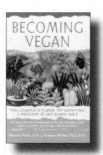

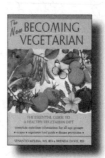

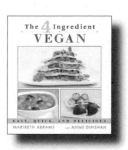

The Natural Vegan Kitchen
Christine Waltermyer
978-1-57067-254-3 $19.95

Becoming Vegan.
Brenda Davis, RD
Vesanto Melina, MS, RD
978-1-57067-103-6 $19.95

The New
Becoming Vegetarian
Vesanto Melina, MS, RD
Brenda Davis, RD
978-1-57067-144-9 $21.95

The 4 Ingredient Vegan
Maribeth Abrams
Anne Dinshah
978-1-57067-232-3 $14.95

Purchase these health titles and cookbooks from your local bookstore
or natural food store,
or you can buy them directly from:

Book Publishing Company • P.O. Box 99
Summertown, TN 38483 • 1-800-695-2241

Please include $3.95 per book for shipping and handling.